Praises for Hot Flashes

Hot Flashes is a funny and entertaining glimpse into the changes women may experience during the menopause transition."

-Rhona Latif M.D., Assistant Clinical Professor,

Medical College of Georgia and NAMS Certified Practitioner

Hot Flashes is a delightful guide for the health and well-being of menopausal women. Robin Gordon serves up an extensive menu of great information and helpful advice peppered with a generous dose of humor.

-Donna Henes

Author of **The Queen of My Self**: *Stepping into Sovereignty in Midlife*

This book is a gem! *Hot Flashes* is a terrific, funny, informative gift to women and those who love them! The resource lists and guides are invaluable. The "Seven Greatest Health Risks for Menopausal Women" is a fantastic, easy-to-read and easy-to-understand guide for women—truly a life-saving tool! Needs to be in every gynecology office!

-Mary L. Lawder,

RN, BSN, FCN

Parish Nurse

Hot Flashes

Marriage and Motherhood in the Menopausal Years

ROBIN L. GORDON

Peaceful Thoughts Press

Disclaimer
The health and medical information provided in this book is not intended to take the place of advice or treatment from your health-care professionals. The author has worked hard to ensure that the information provided in this book is timely, accurate and helpful. This information should not be considered medical advice. One should consult with her health-care provider. The information provided is for general reference purposes only. Always obtain advice from your physician or other qualified health-care provider before starting any new treatment.

Published by
Peaceful Thoughts Press
Marietta, Georgia
www.hotflashesforwomen.com

Publishing Support by:
Booklogix Publishing Services
Alpharetta, Georgia

ISBN 978-1-81005-013-5

Introduction

A few years ago, I involuntarily landed in a place called Poz, short for perimenopause. Similar to Dorothy who, along with her entire house, made an unintended visit to Oz after a whirlwind storm, the events that ultimately led me to my good witch, Dr. GYNda, were equally unexpected and unsettling, to say the least. Dr. GYNda advised me that I wasn't in Kansas anymore - talk about confirming the obvious - and that things were going to be quite different here in the land of Poz for now and ever more.

Unlike Dorothy's journey, mine was a one-way trip and unfortunately, a strange dream from which I would not eventually awake. Nor was there any great 'Wizard of Poz' to award a certificate of courage, a bigger heart, or a sharper brain. Similarly though, there were fields of poppy causing my fatigue and there were winged monkeys, in the form of hormonal shifts, triggering my night sweats, weight gain, irritability, brain fuzz, and a general feeling of being off-center.

Although the good witch assured me that this was all normal, my journey was not without its detours and roadblocks. Complicating matters further, I found myself with a continually changing navigation system that left me feeling as if I were playing a high-speed video game without adequate control over the joystick. Then, an amazing thing happened.

While attempting to navigate this strange new land with a husband and teen-ager in tow, I began to have 'out-of-mind' experiences - I'm not kidding! I began to see myself in a cartoon, and suddenly, it all seemed hilarious to me. I thought to myself, "This is a new kind of HRT, Hilarious Response Therapy, without the side effects!"

Inbetween the hot flashes (if you're not sure whether or not you're having them, then you're not having them yet, trust me), I began to chronicle these humorous moments into a book with the intent of sharing them with women who may need their own dose of HRT as they undertake their deeply personal and often unsettling journeys.

In addition to journaling the events, I thought to provide a comprehensive chart entitled The Seven Greatest Health Risks for Menopausal Women, listing the most common health risks, associated symptoms, screening tools, and best preventative measures. You will also discover a Menopause Glossary of Terms and Index of Resources so you will not have to undertake this journey alone.

I hope that as you hit those bumpy and unfamiliar roads in Poz, HOT FLASHES will be a source of humor and information that helps you find the courage you need to face this strange new place, the intelligence to make sense of your changing biological processes, and the heart to help guide you back to your own beloved "Kansas".

I want to offer my heartfelt appreciation to my family and friends who hosed me down (several times mind you) when I was too hot to handle! Special thanks to my cartoonist, Matt Hawkins, an extraordinary illustrator who gave shape to my visions so that others may fully appreciate them. Even after sharing voluminous visions with him, Matt never questioned any of my 'observations' - a very smart way to negotiate a perimenopausal woman!

May your journey through "Poz" afford you an open mind and an open heart for this much-needed book of humor and may you faithfully survive marriage and motherhood along the way.

Stay cool, and see you on the other side!

Robin L. Gordon

Acknowledgements

It is with deep gratitude that I acknowledge John Fayad, Literary Coach, who provided continual encouragement and helpful editing at the outset of the publishing process. I also wish to thank Dr. Rhonda Latif, Assistant Clinical Professor at the Medical College of Georgia and National Association of Menopause Society Certified Practitioner in Gynecology, for fine tuning the content editing.

It is with eternal appreciation and love that I acknowledge my husband, Sam, who has patiently witnessed many of my "hot flashes" and continues to provide the love and support I need on a daily basis. Fortunately, he is NOT the one depicted in this book! I'd also like to send a big "Woo-hoo" and lots of love and appreciation to my daughter, Laura, who weathered many of the menopausal storms with me and emerged, a beautiful, loving, and very cool young lady.

Table of Contents

Chapter One: Introduction to the Menopausal Years 1

Chapter Two: Marriage & Menopause 25

Chapter Three: Motherhood & Menopause 35

Chapter Four: Generational Differences 45

Chapter Five: Preventative Maintenance 55

Appendices: 71

The Seven Greatest Health Risks Chart 73

Body Mass Index Information & Chart 75

Menopause Glossary of Terms 77

Resources for Women 81

About The Author 93

Chapter One

Introduction to the Menopausal Years

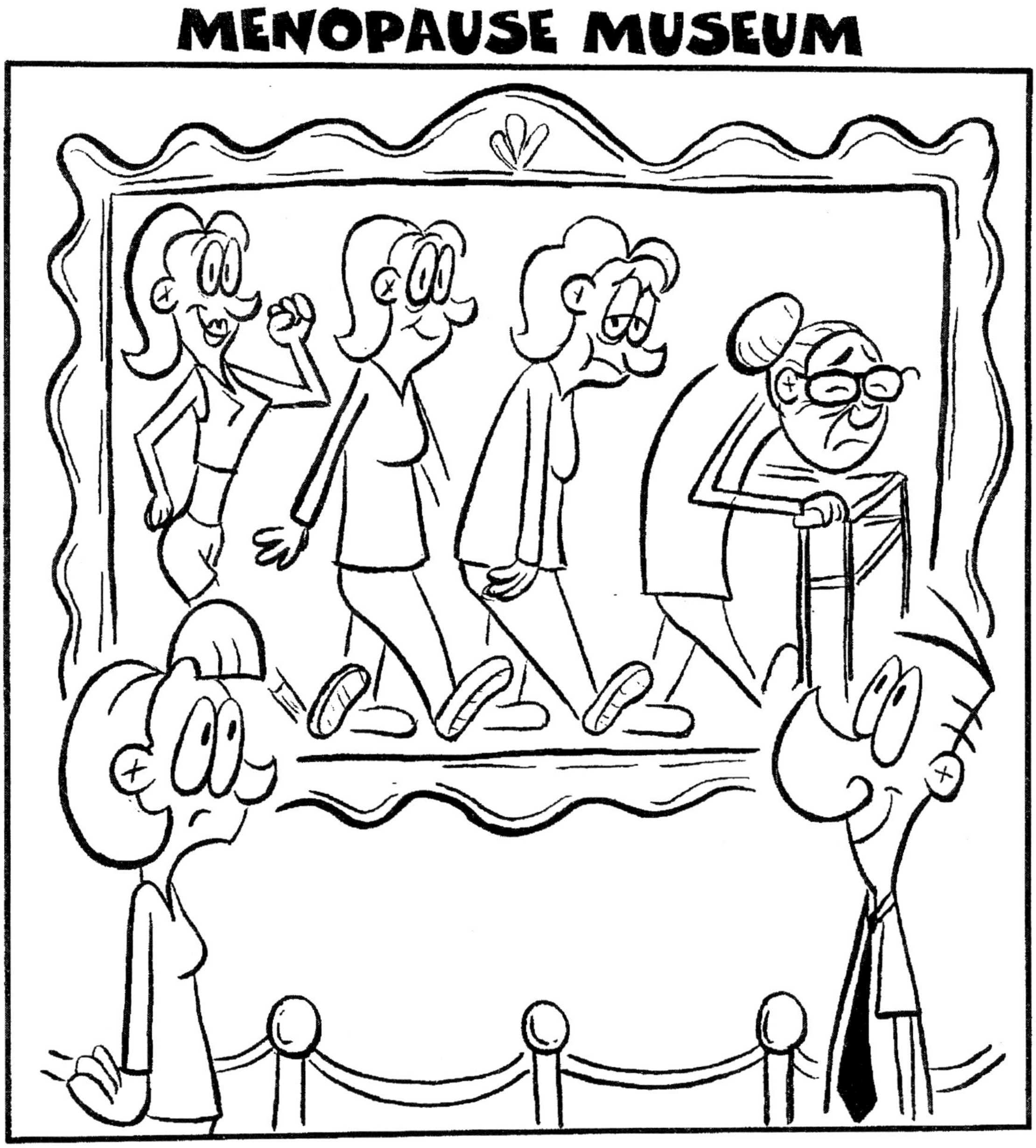

At about mid-point in a woman's life, between forty and sixty years of age, physical changes begin to occur, both internally and externally.

IS SHE OR ISN'T SHE?

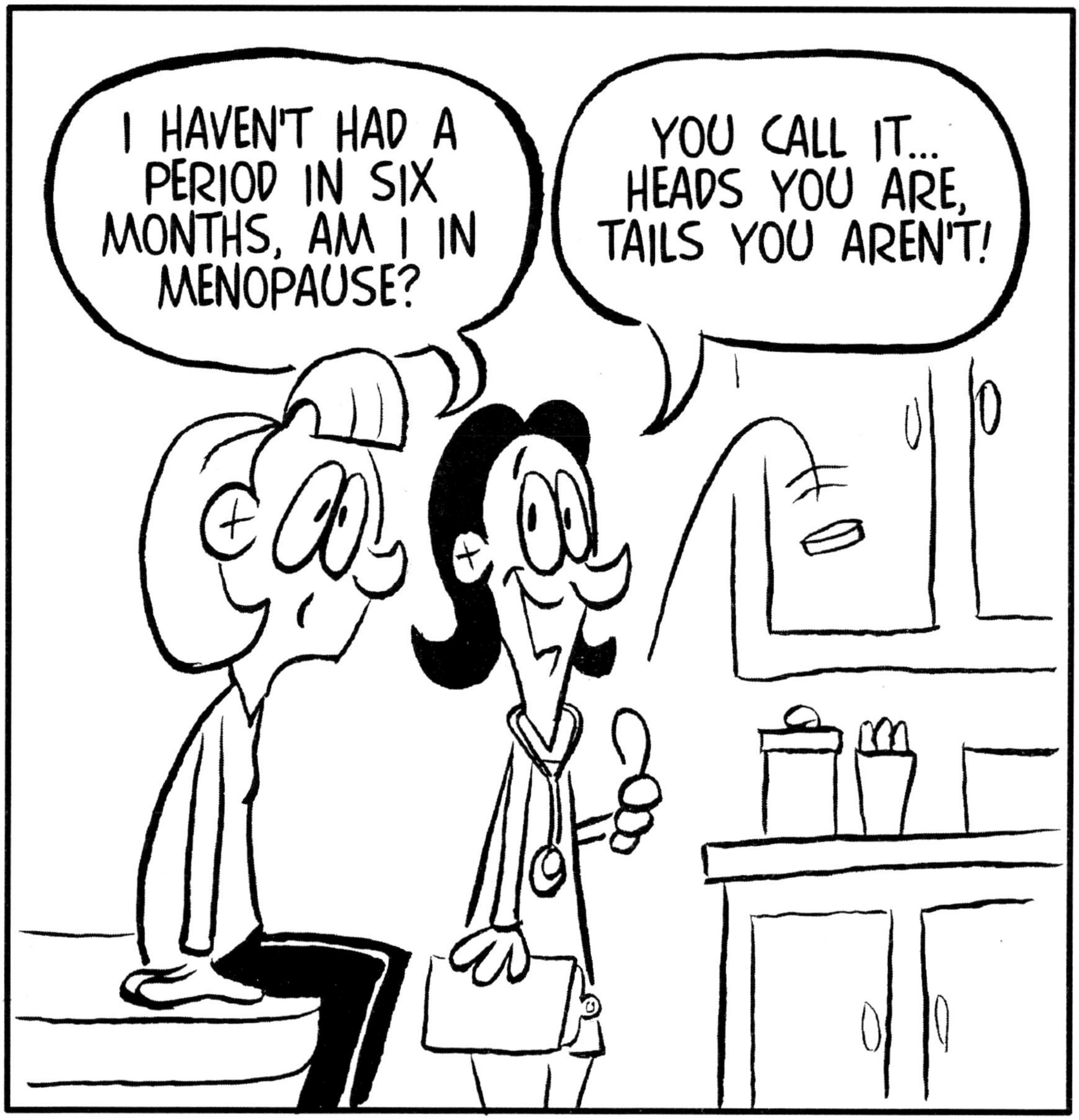
I HAVEN'T HAD A PERIOD IN SIX MONTHS, AM I IN MENOPAUSE?
YOU CALL IT... HEADS YOU ARE, TAILS YOU AREN'T!

Some women begin to notice a change in their routine menstrual periods, ranging from less frequency and lighter flow to greater frequency and heavier flow.

ETCH A SKETCH

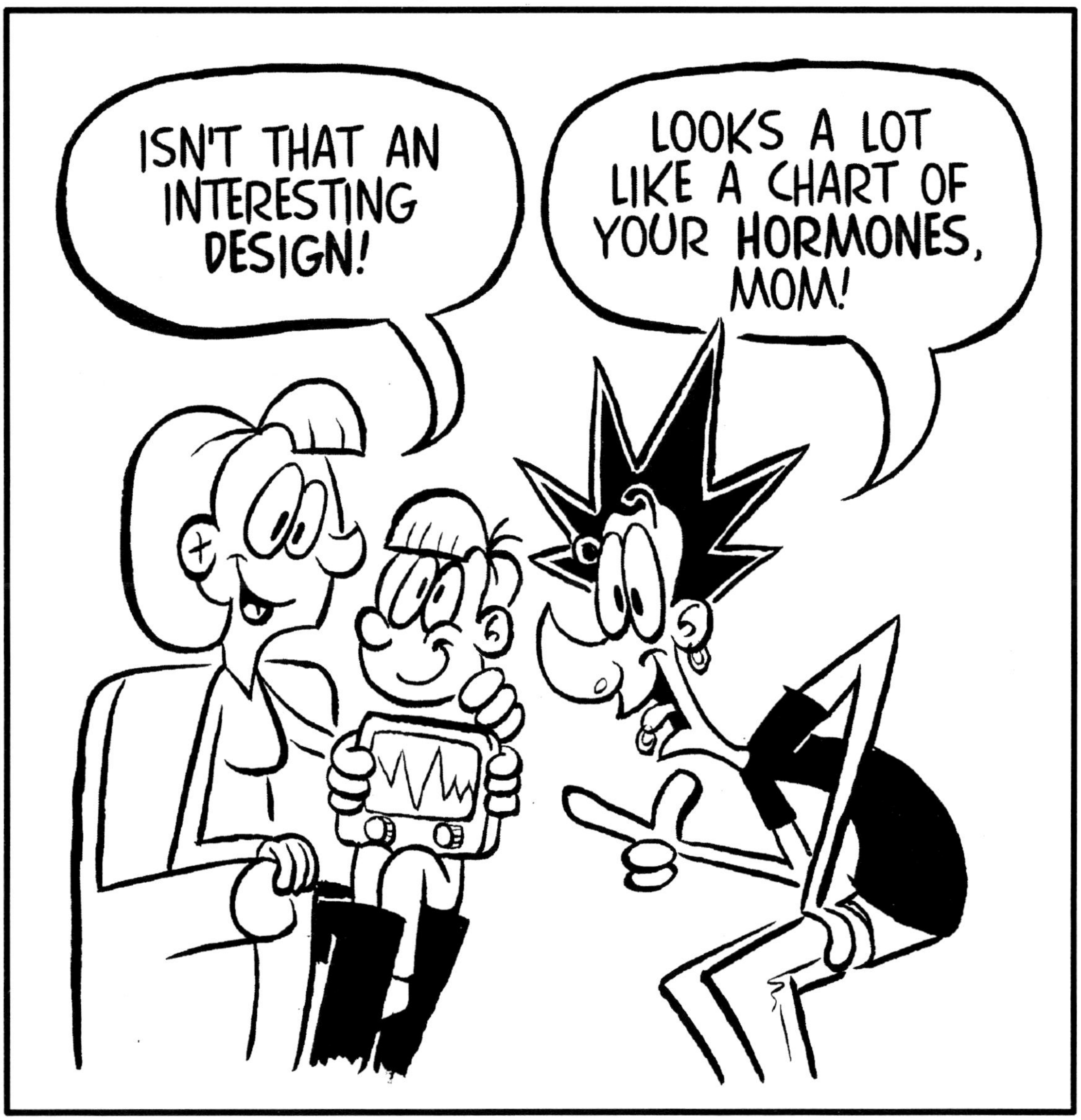
ISN'T THAT AN INTERESTING DESIGN!
LOOKS A LOT LIKE A CHART OF YOUR HORMONES, MOM!

The cause of these changes is fluctuating hormone levels, specifically estrogen, progesterone, and testosterone.

MID-LIFE BABY BLUES

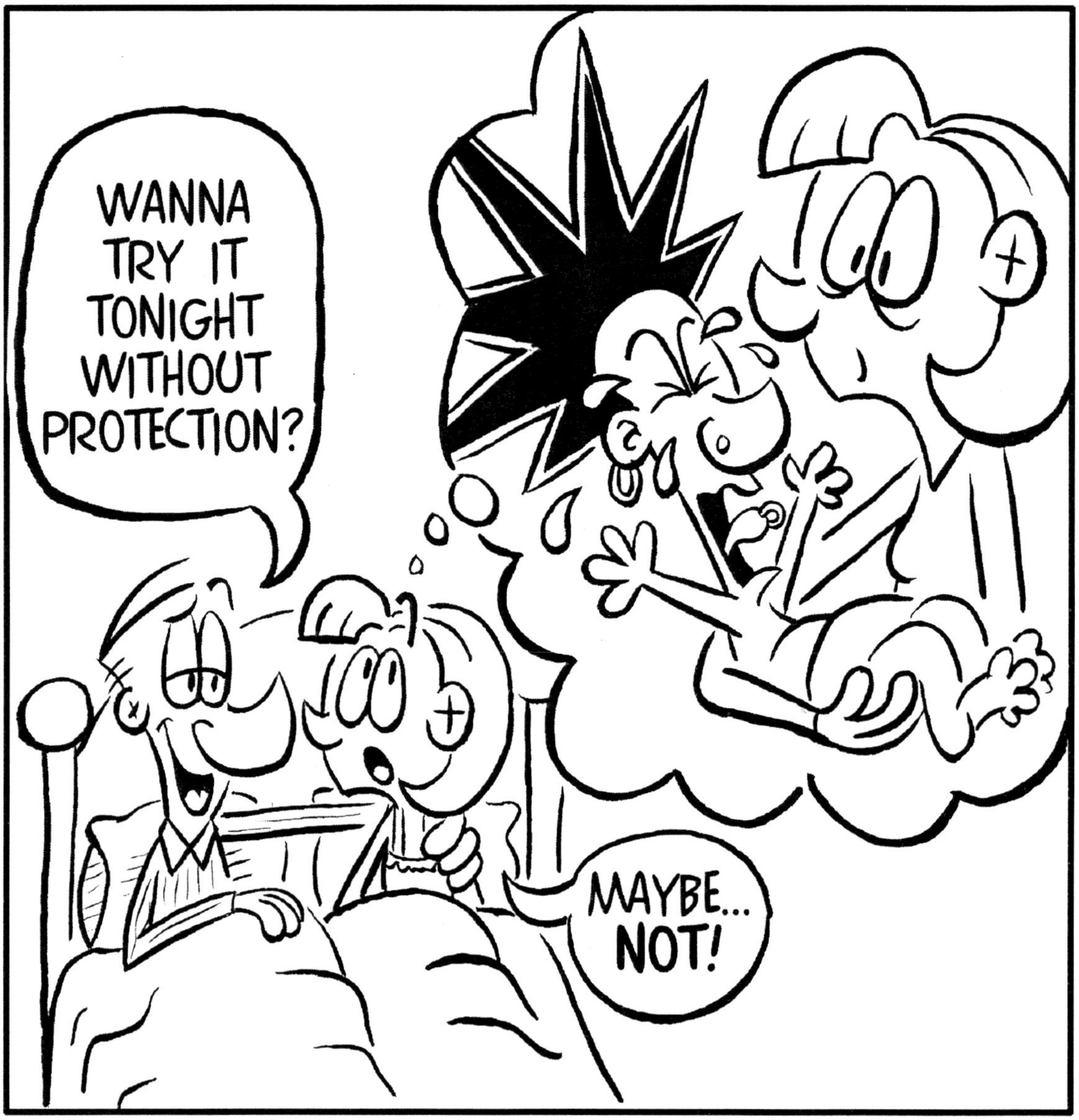

The ovaries begin to shut down the process of producing hormones to signal the release of a monthly egg. Until this function completely stops, a woman may still become pregnant.

MENOPAUSAL CYCLE

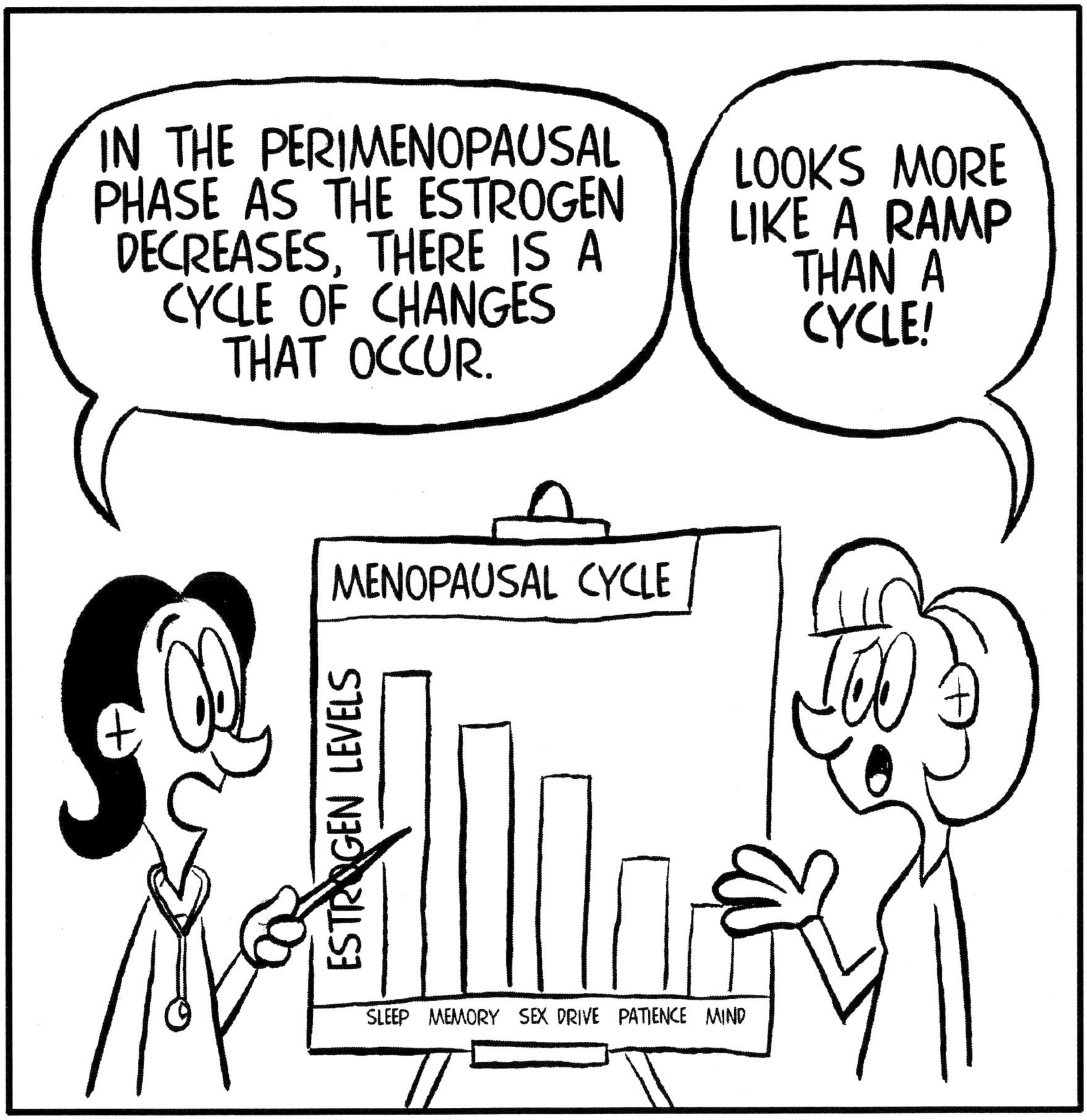

The first phase of these changes called Perimenopause, may last from four to six years. As the estrogen levels decrease during this time, many other body systems may also become affected.

OFF THE CHART

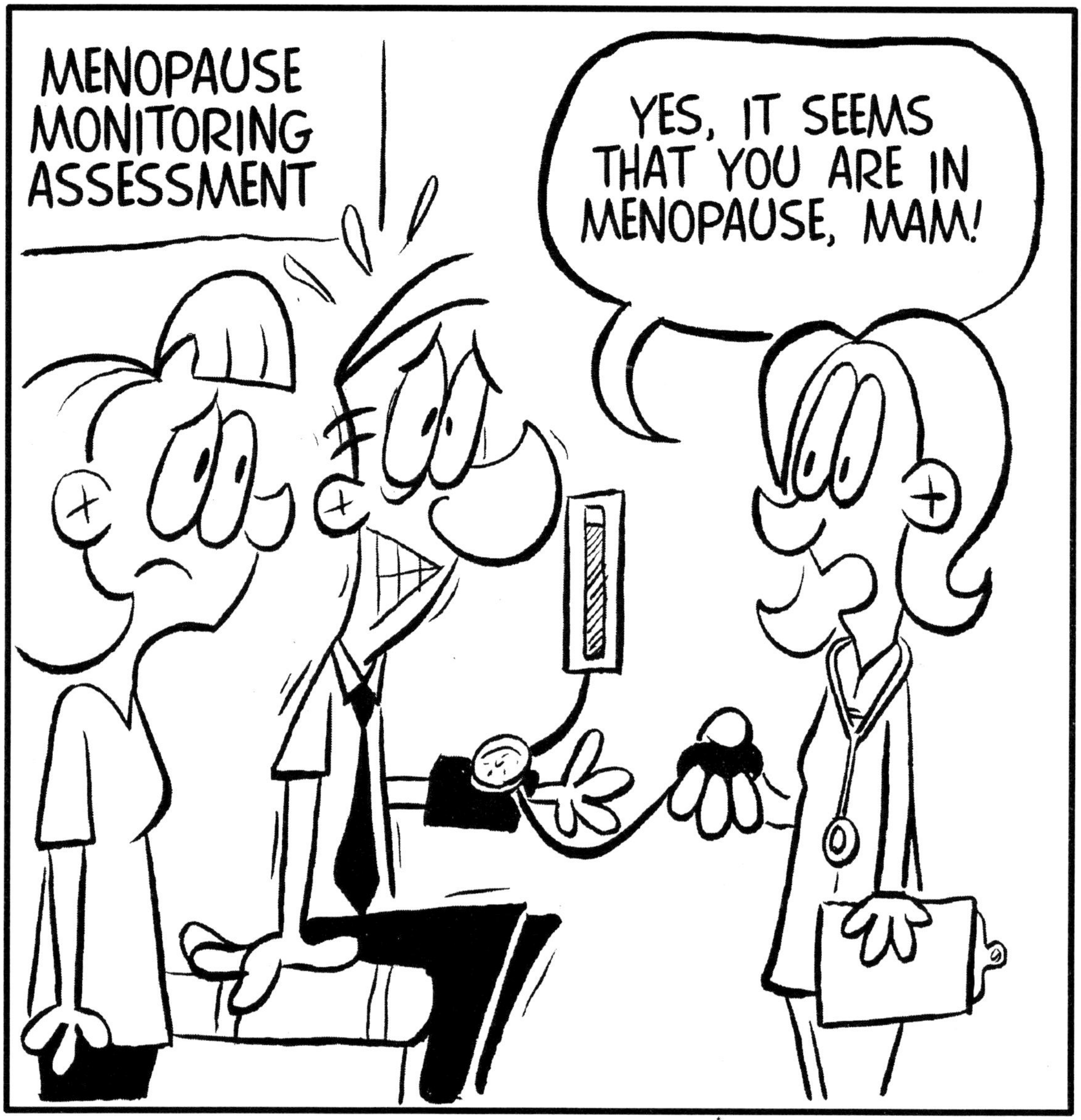
MENOPAUSE
MONITORING
ASSESSMENT
YES, IT SEEMS
THAT YOU ARE IN
MENOPAUSE, MAM!

A woman is considered to be in menopause when twelve consecutive months have passed without her experiencing a menstrual period.

HRT ONLINE

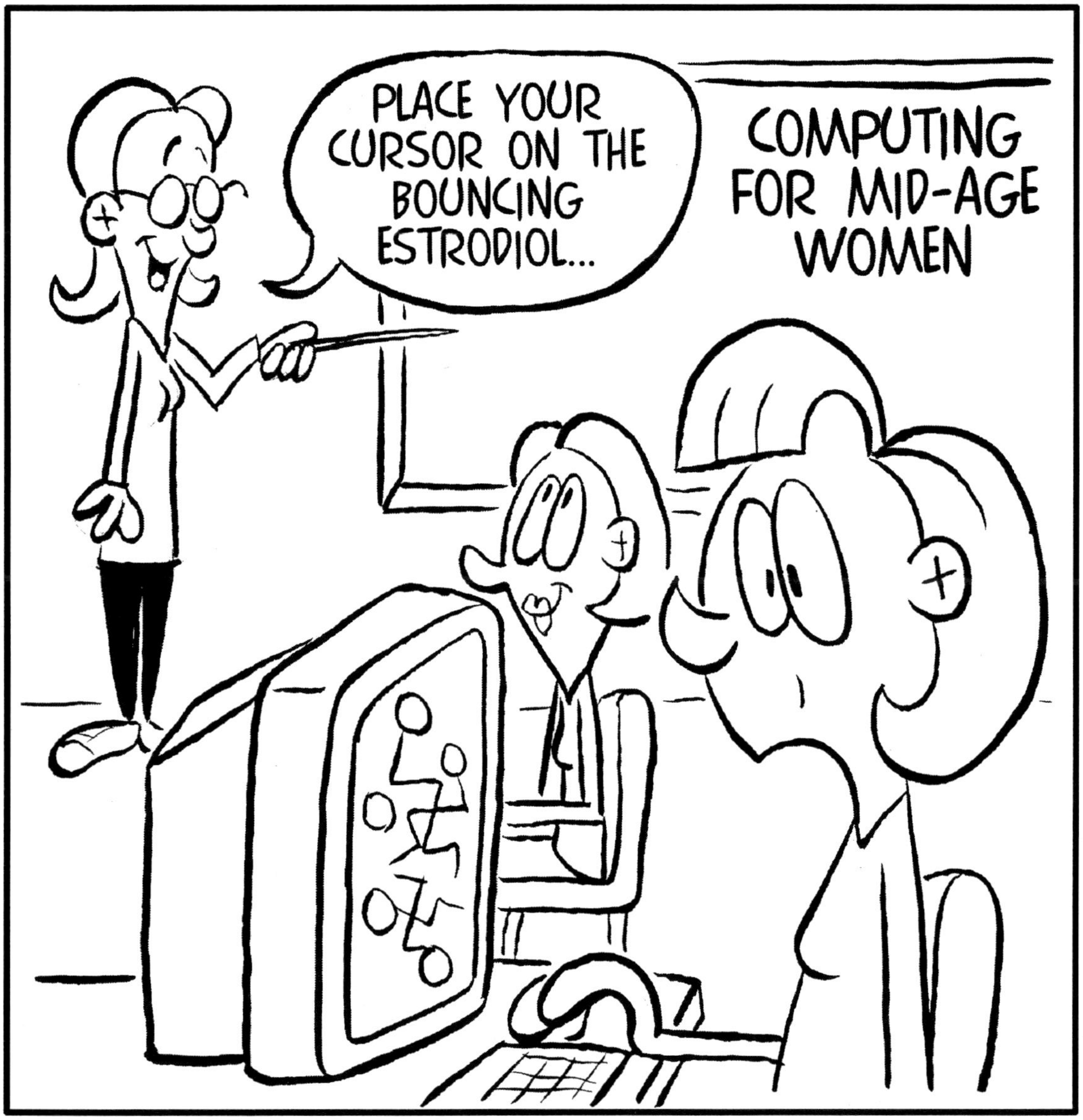
PLACE YOUR CURSOR ON THE BOUNCING ESTRODIOL...
COMPUTING FOR MID-AGE WOMEN

If a woman is taking birth control pills, it may be difficult to determine if twelve consecutive months have passed naturally without a menstrual period.

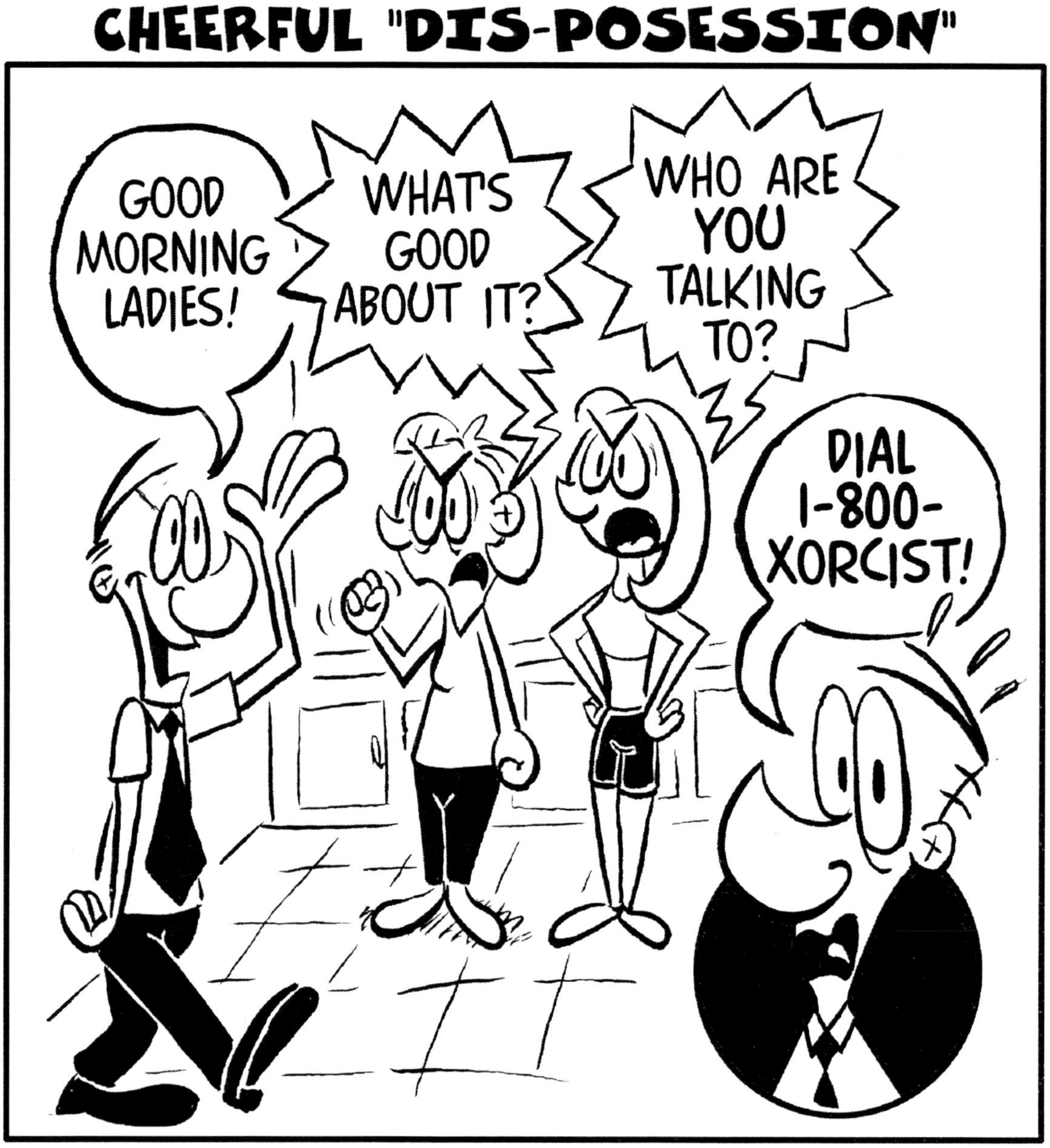
CHEERFUL "DIS-POSESSION"
GOOD MORNING LADIES!
WHAT'S GOOD ABOUT IT?
WHO ARE YOU TALKING TO?
DIAL 1-800-XORCIST!

The hormonal shifts may affect temperament and women may experience greater moodiness for no apparent reason.

KOOL AID

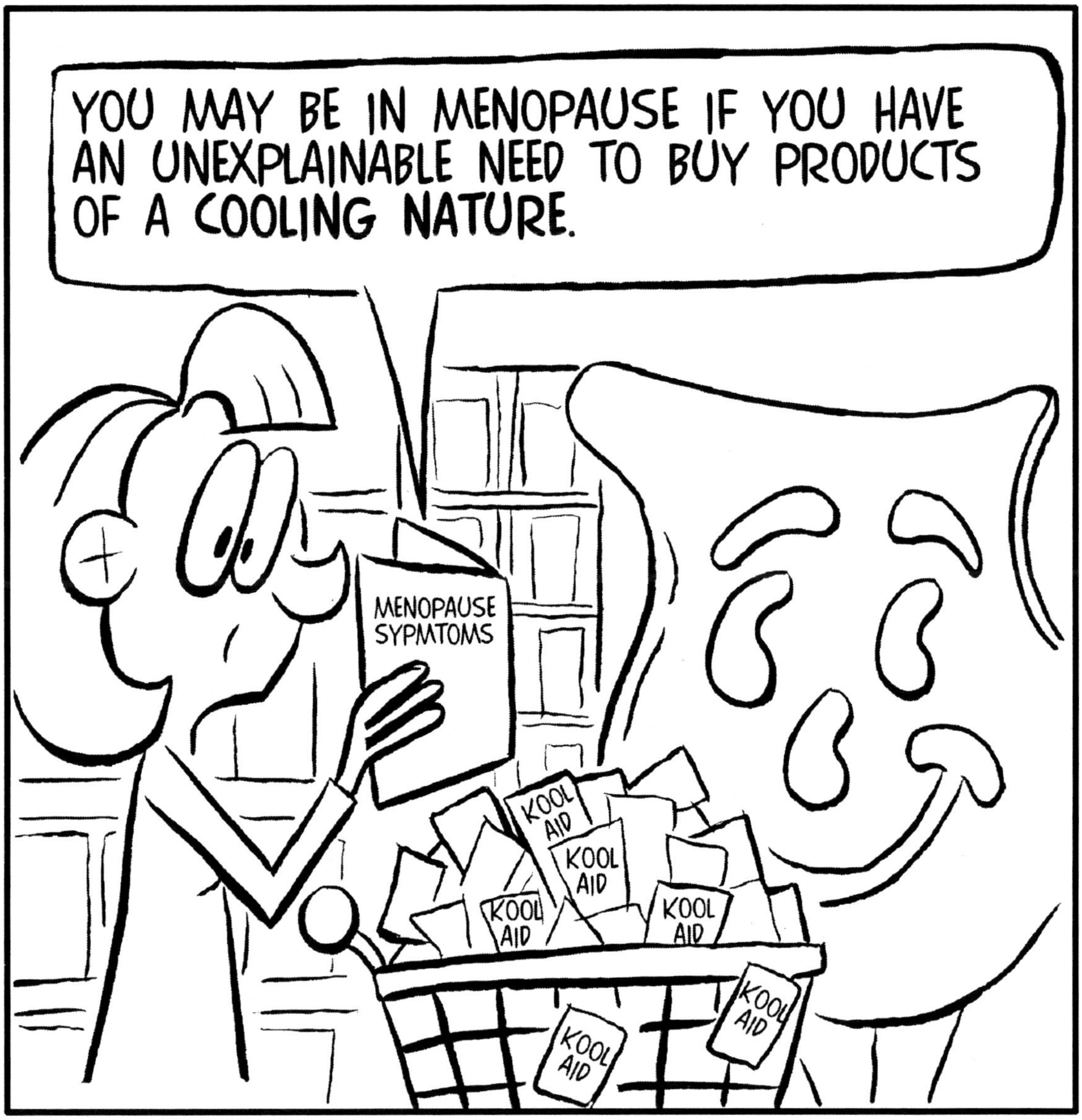

Some women experience an abrupt increase in their body temperature without warning. This heat wave is called a "hot flash".

THE BIG CHILL

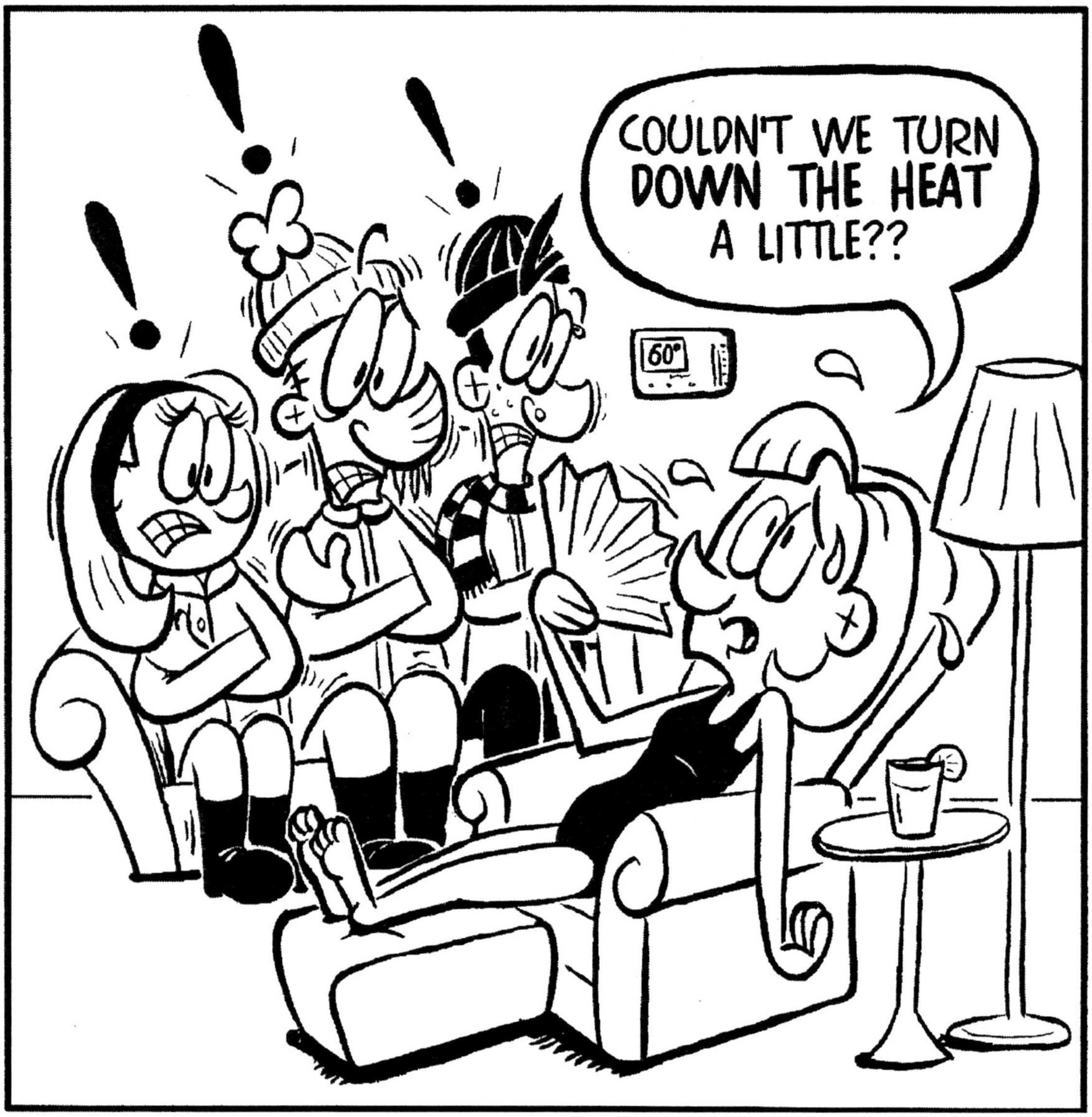

You may be experiencing hot flashes if you no longer need to heat your home in the winter.

FOUNTAIN OF YOUTH

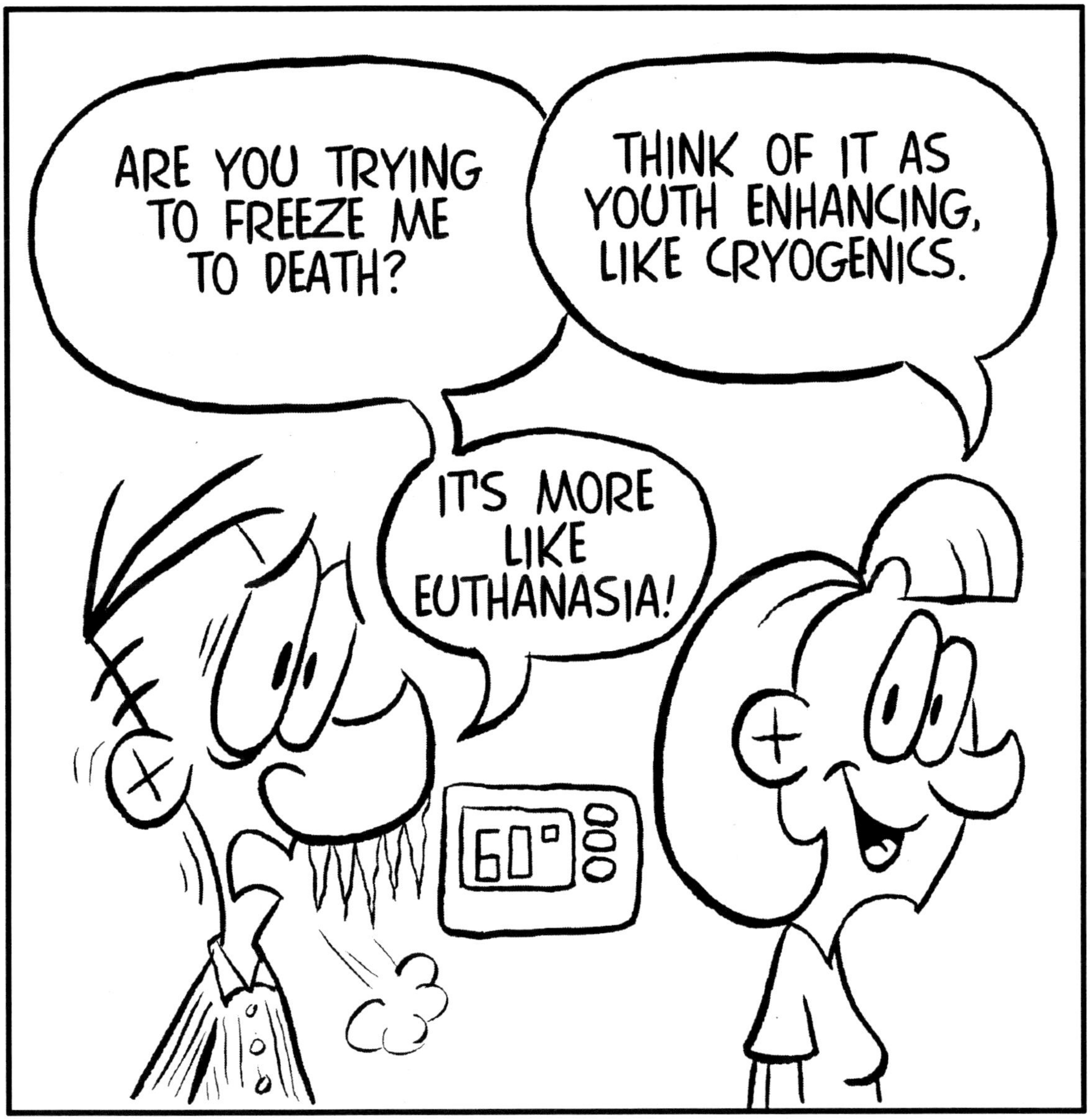
ARE YOU TRYING TO FREEZE ME TO DEATH?
THINK OF IT AS YOUTH ENHANCING, LIKE CRYOGENICS.
IT'S MORE LIKE EUTHANASIA!
60°

On the other hand, your changing climate needs may create conflict among family members.

PUDDLE HUDDLE

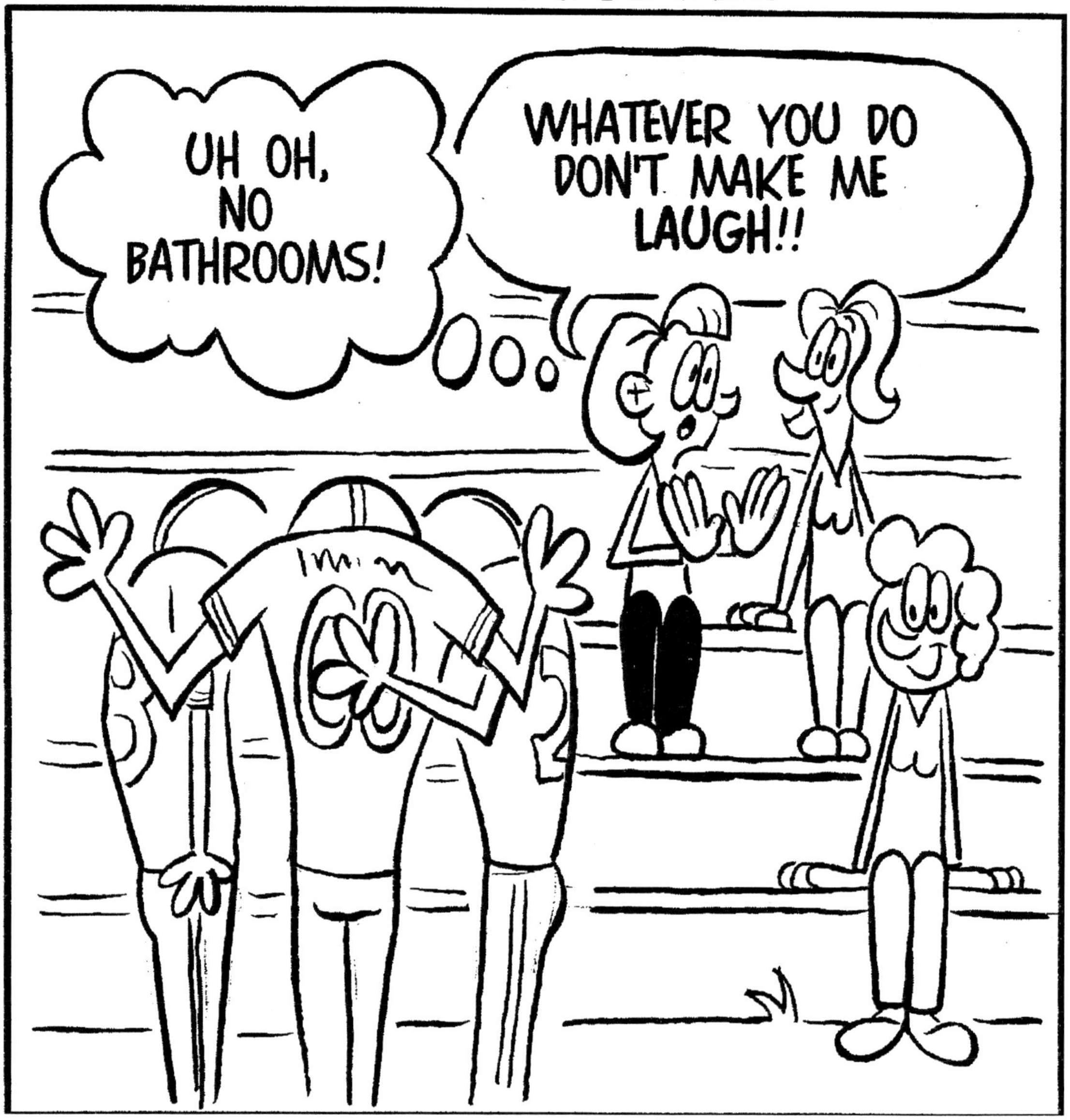
UH OH,
NO
BATHROOMS!
WHATEVER YOU DO
DON'T MAKE ME
LAUGH!!

Some women may experience urine leakage due to changing estrogen levels. Sanitary pads: never leave home without them!

HAIR TODAY, GONE TOMORROW

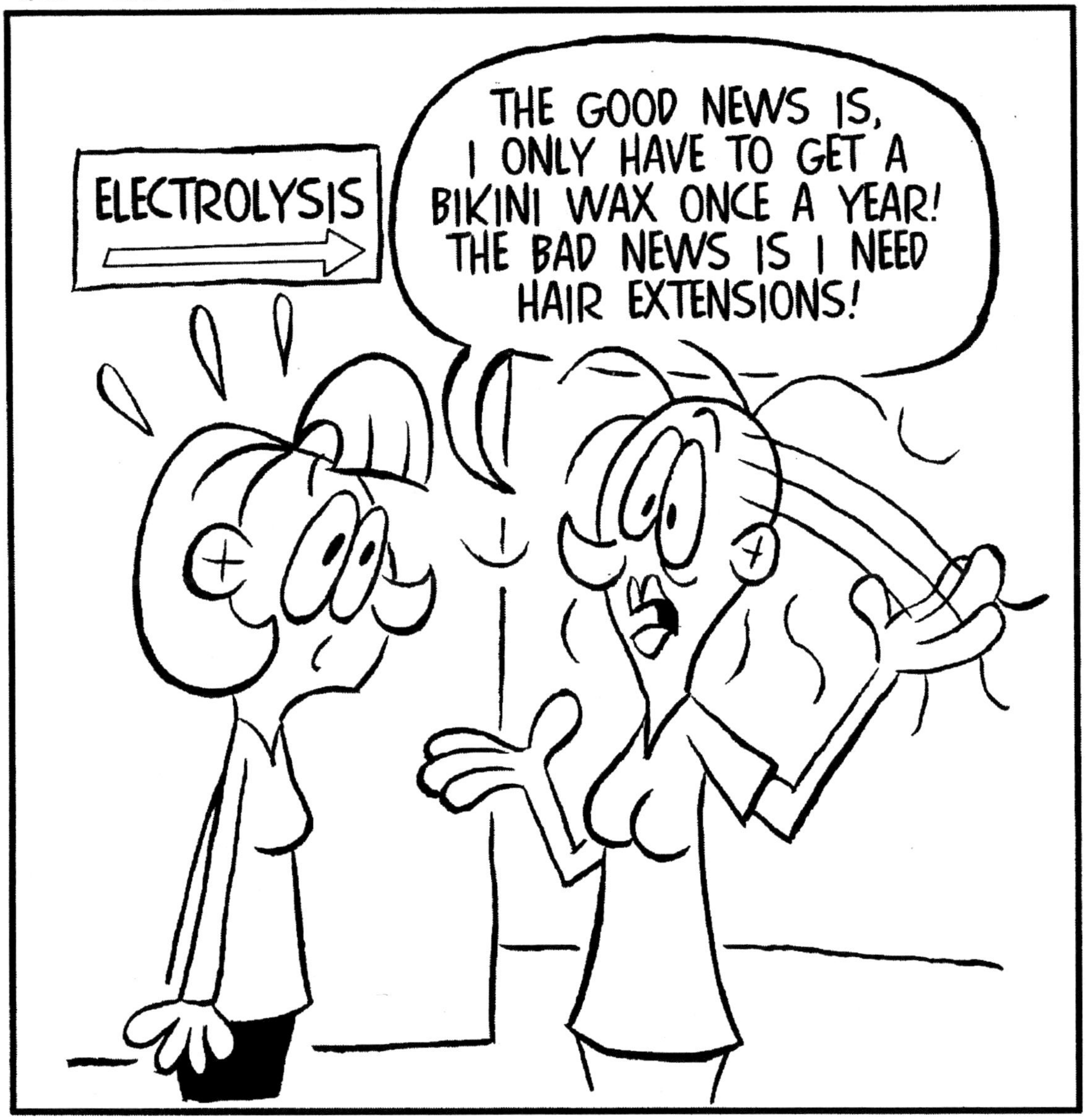
ELECTROLYSIS
THE GOOD NEWS IS, I ONLY HAVE TO GET A BIKINI WAX ONCE A YEAR! THE BAD NEWS IS I NEED HAIR EXTENSIONS!

While some women experience thinning of the hair on their head, follicles may appear on other areas of their face. More lip wax and a new pair of tweezers are strongly recommended.

SHAPING UP

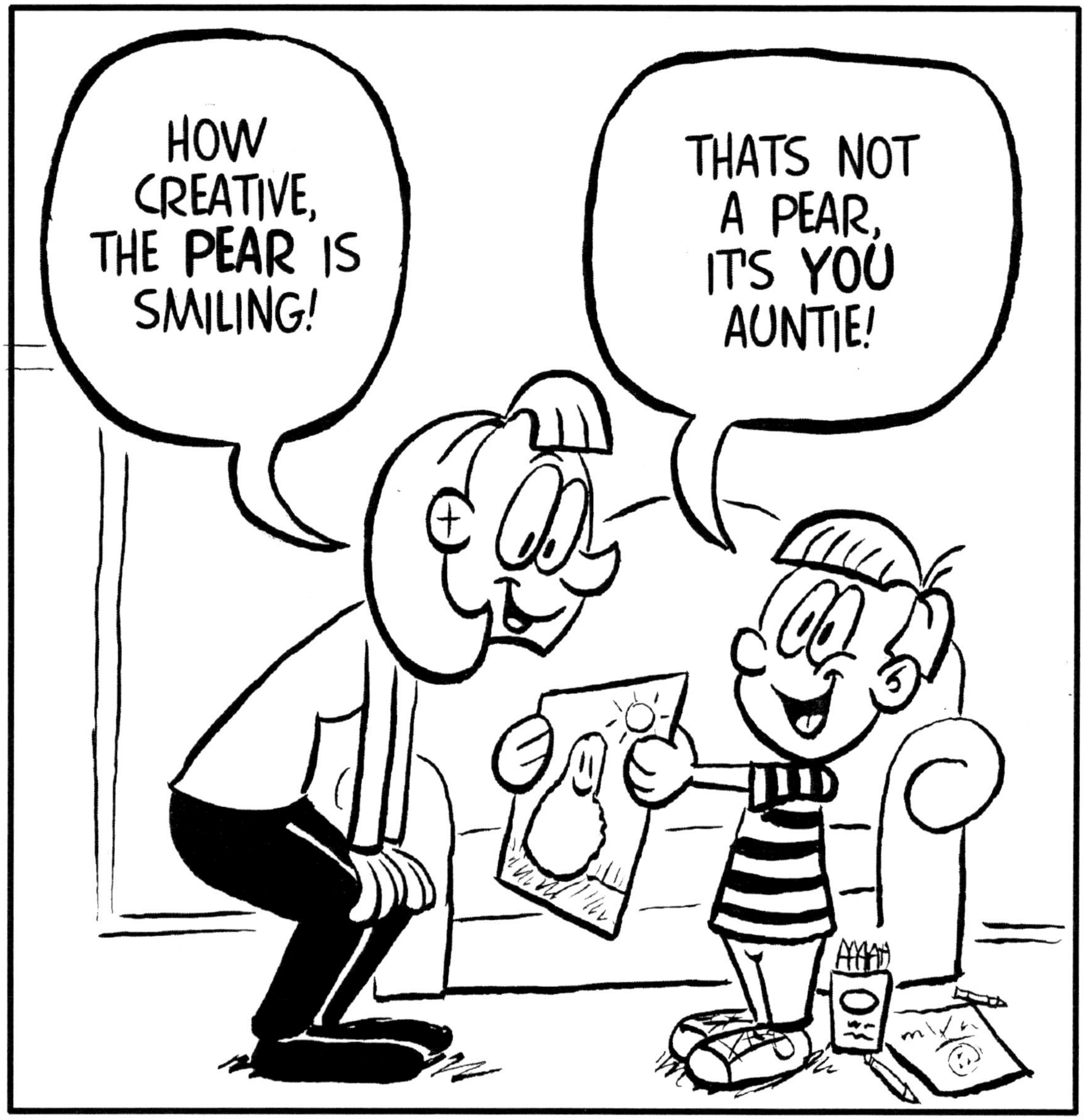
HOW CREATIVE, THE PEAR IS SMILING!
THATS NOT A PEAR, IT'S YOU AUNTIE!

Women often notice a change in their body shape during this period. As the body ages, metabolism slows down due to a decrease in lean muscle mass. Physical activity, especially resistance training, can increase lean muscle mass which increases resting metabolism. Many women consider weight loss plans, changes in exercise regimes, and other creative ways of toning their bodies.

WOMEN IN BLACK

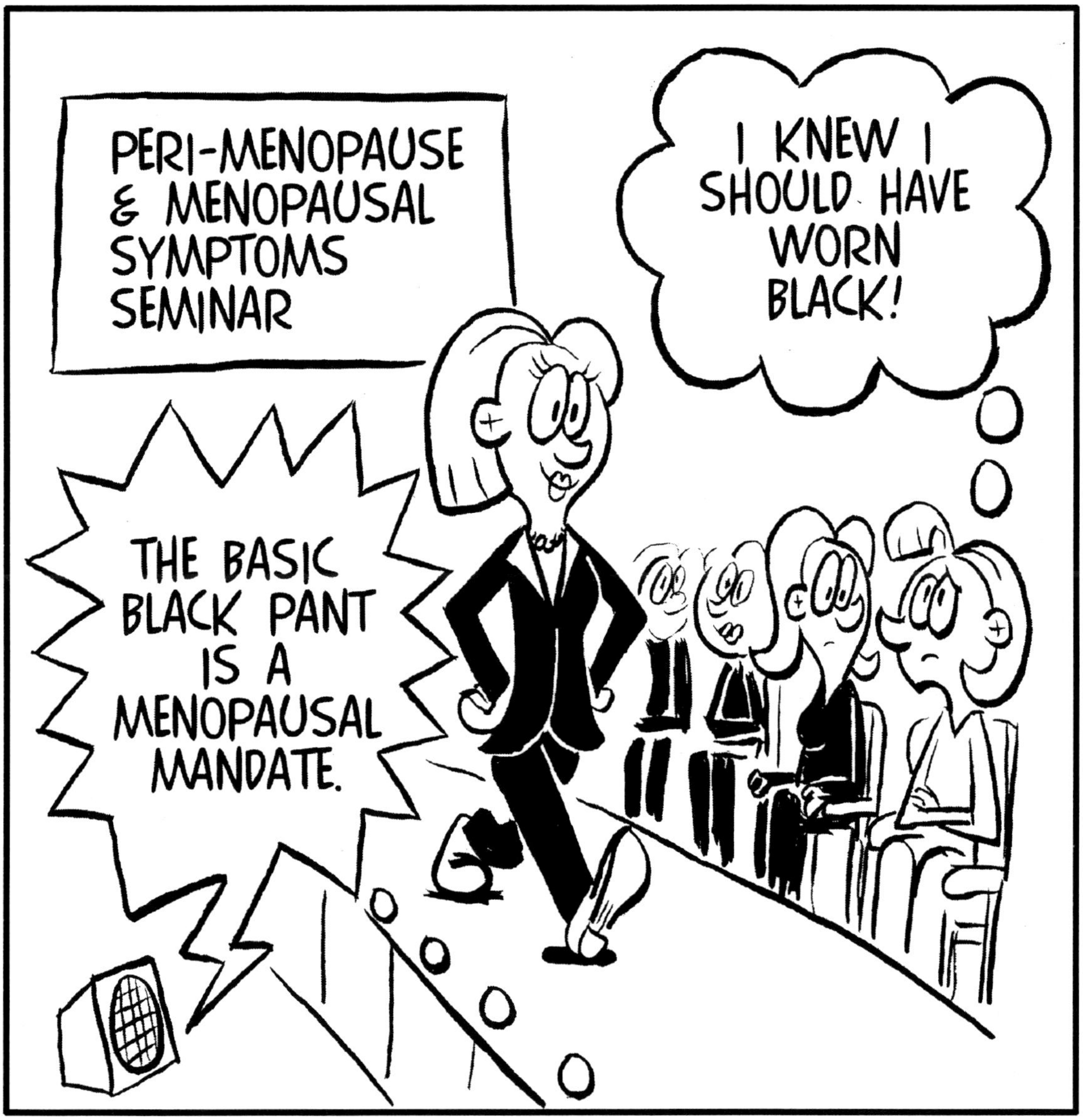
PERI-MENOPAUSE & MENOPAUSAL SYMPTOMS SEMINAR
I KNEW I SHOULD HAVE WORN BLACK!
THE BASIC BLACK PANT IS A MENOPAUSAL MANDATE.

Other women choose to revamp their wardrobe to complement their new body shapes.

NIGHTWEAR NUISANCE

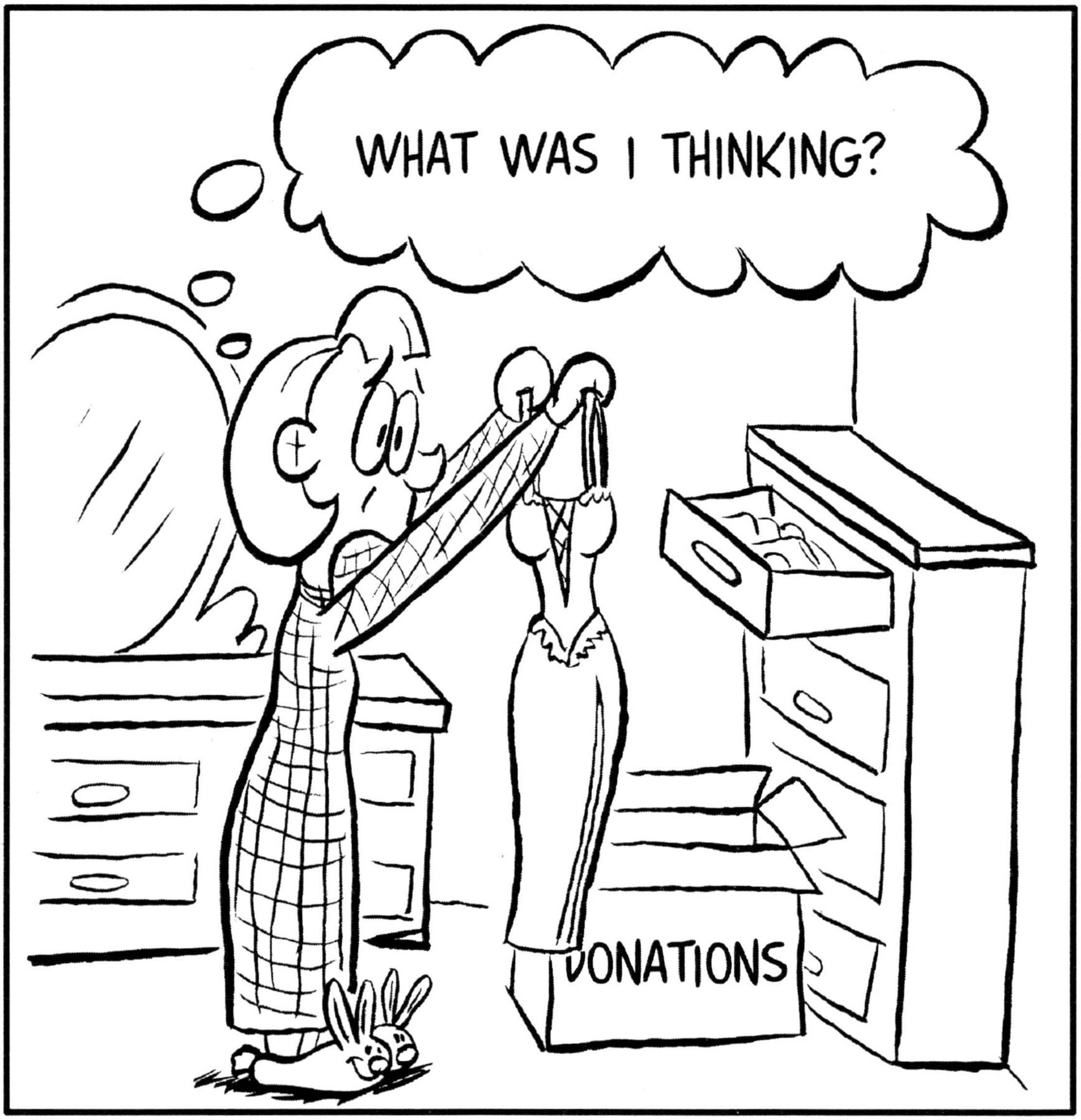

For some women, sexual desire will decrease in conjunction with hormonal changes.

GOOD VIBRATIONS

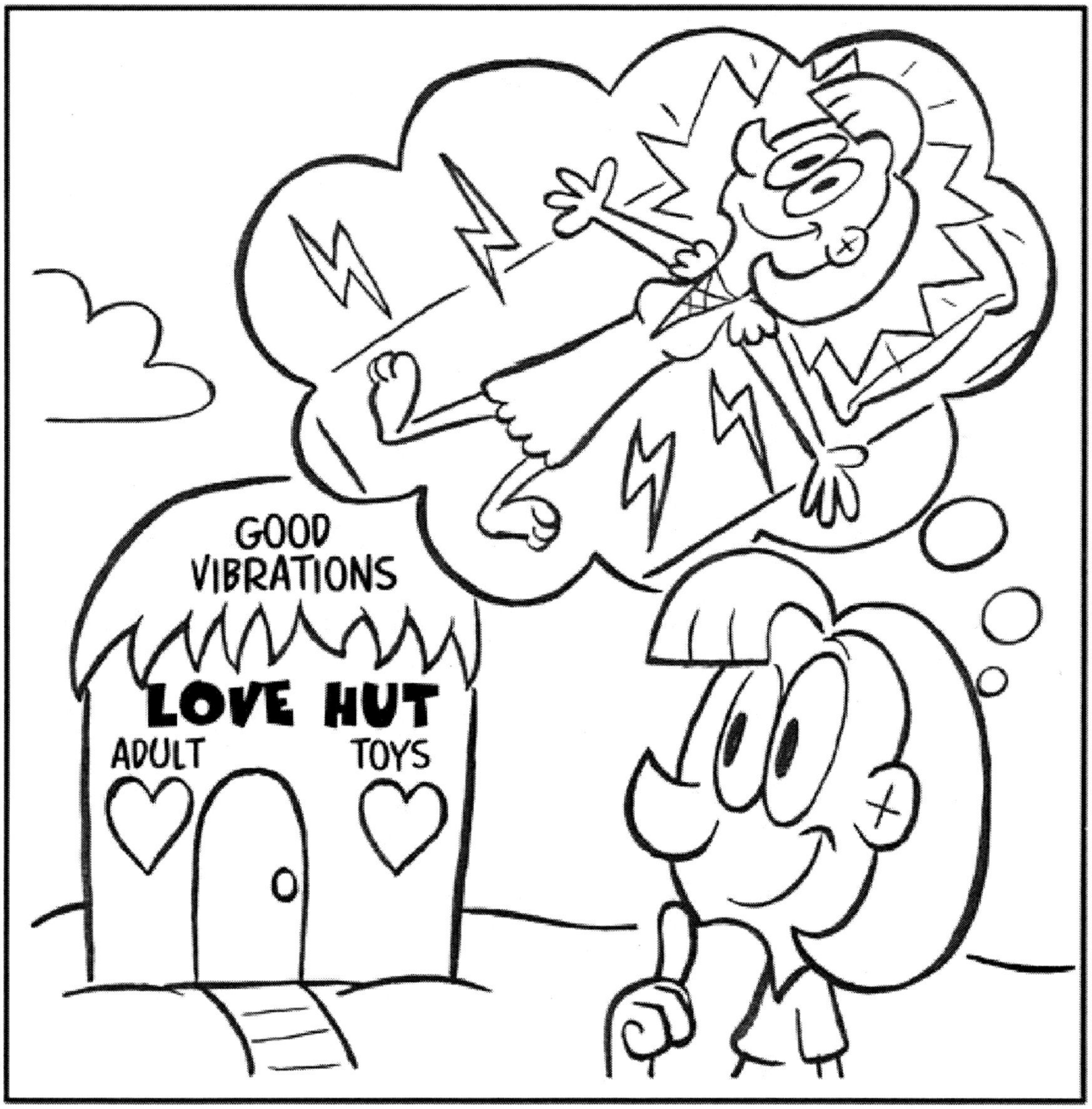

Many women seek out new ways to stimulate their desire and make sexual relations more enjoyable. Vaginal lubricants and power tools may prove helpful.

CALENDAR GIRLS REVISITED

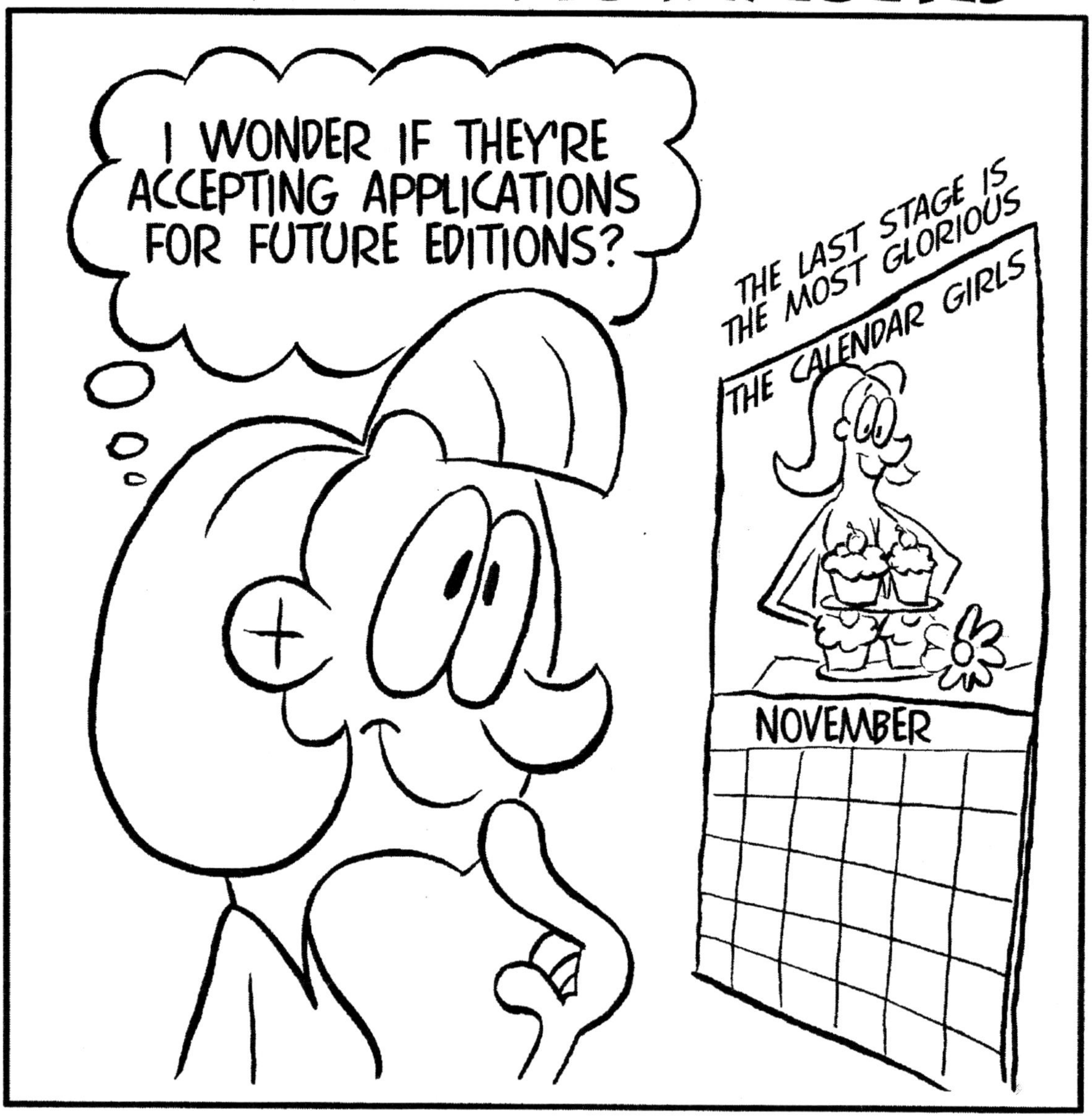
I WONDER IF THEY'RE ACCEPTING APPLICATIONS FOR FUTURE EDITIONS?
THE LAST STAGE IS THE MOST GLORIOUS
THE CALENDAR GIRLS
NOVEMBER

For many women, this is a sexually liberating time, which may also increase desire, as they are no longer worried about pregnancy.

SLEEPLESS NIGHTS

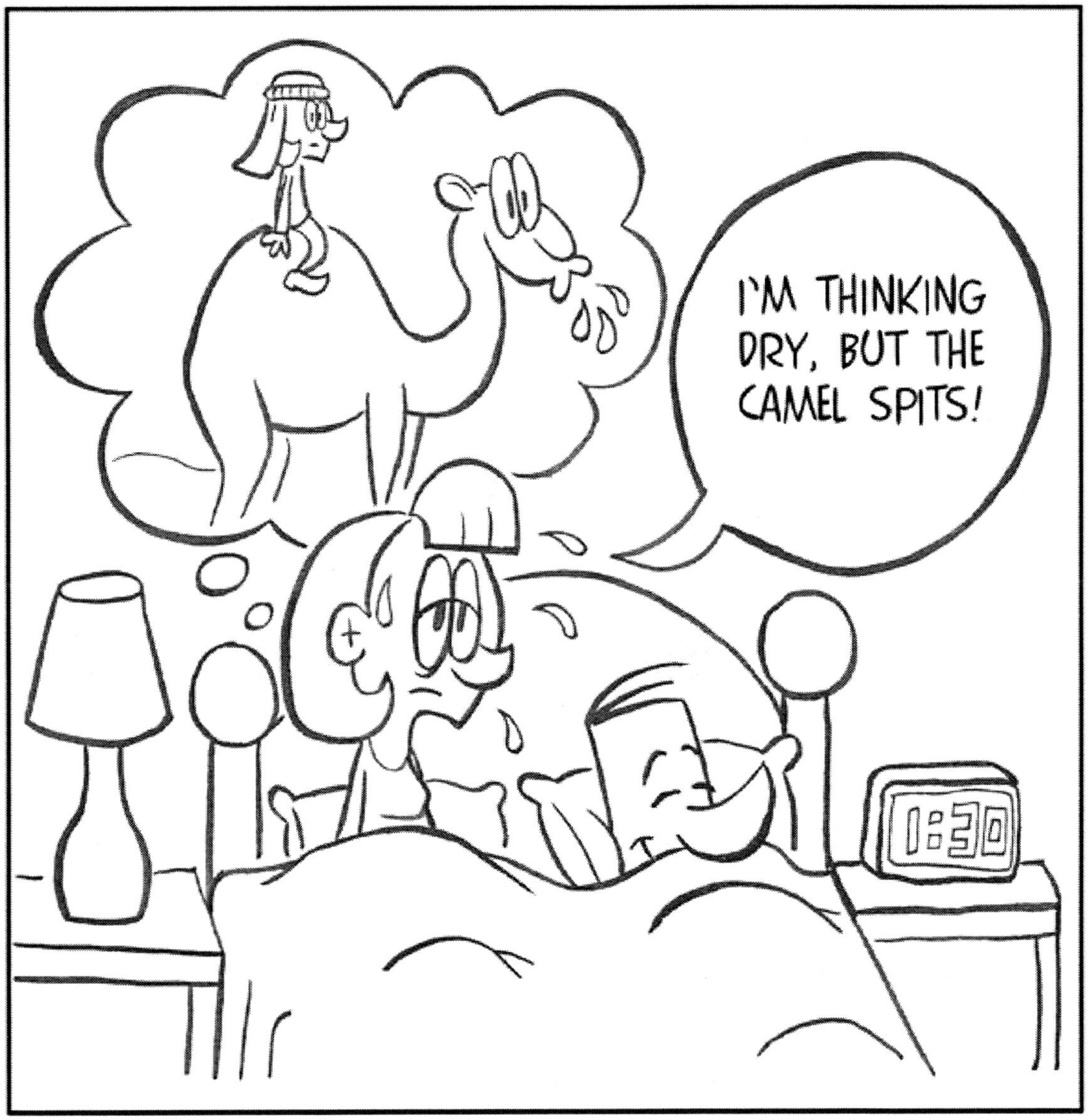

Sleep disturbances and night sweats may become common occurrences. Many women seek out light-weight nightwear with a wicking capacity to keep them dry and comfortable. Setting a glass of cool water by the bed table is a good idea.

THE AGE OF ENLIGHTENMENT

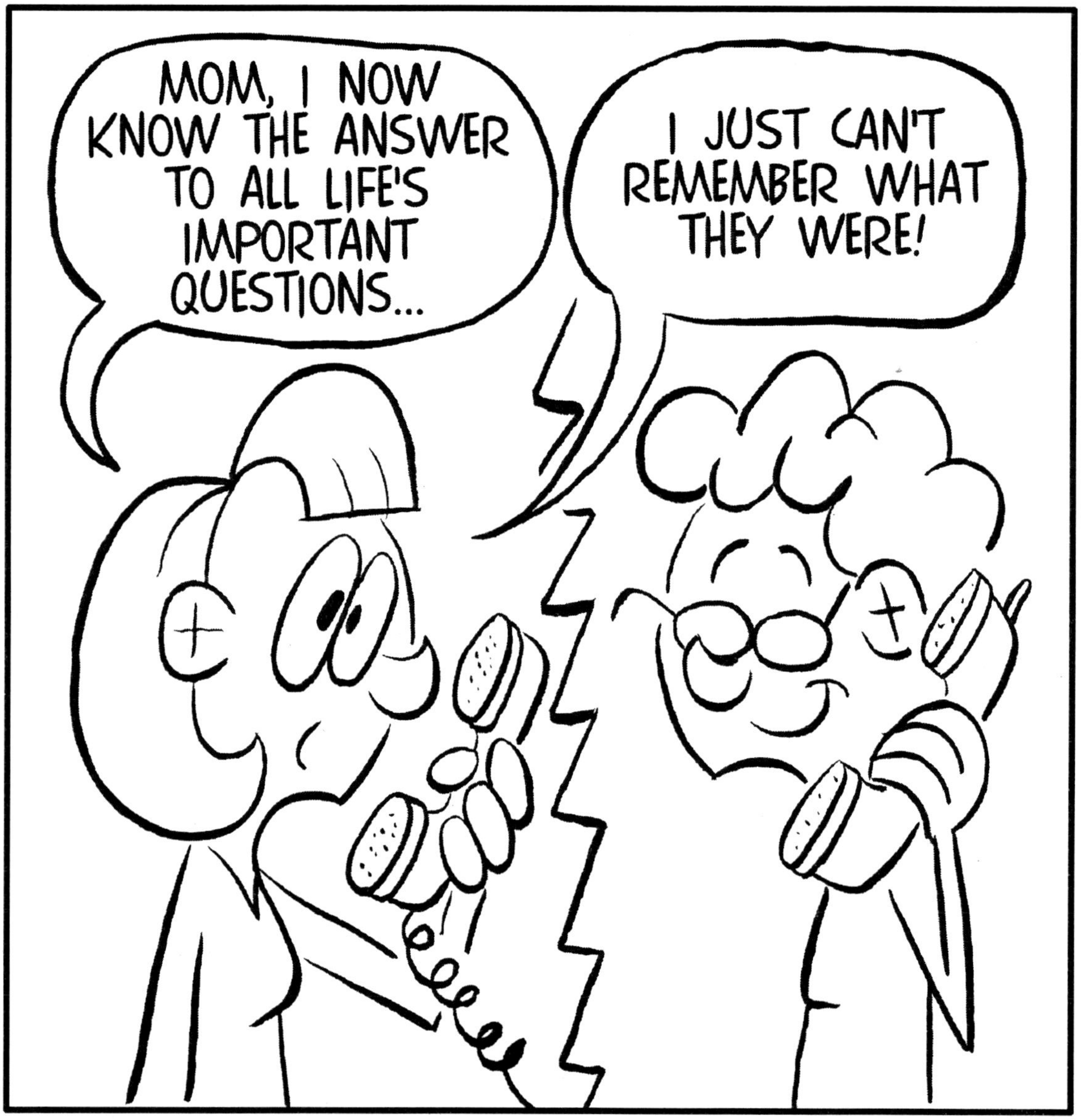
MOM, I NOW KNOW THE ANSWER TO ALL LIFE'S IMPORTANT QUESTIONS...
I JUST CAN'T REMEMBER WHAT THEY WERE!

Hormonal changes and lack of consistent sleep may begin to affect memory. Physical exercise, especially aerobic activity, is associated with helping to enhance memory as we age.

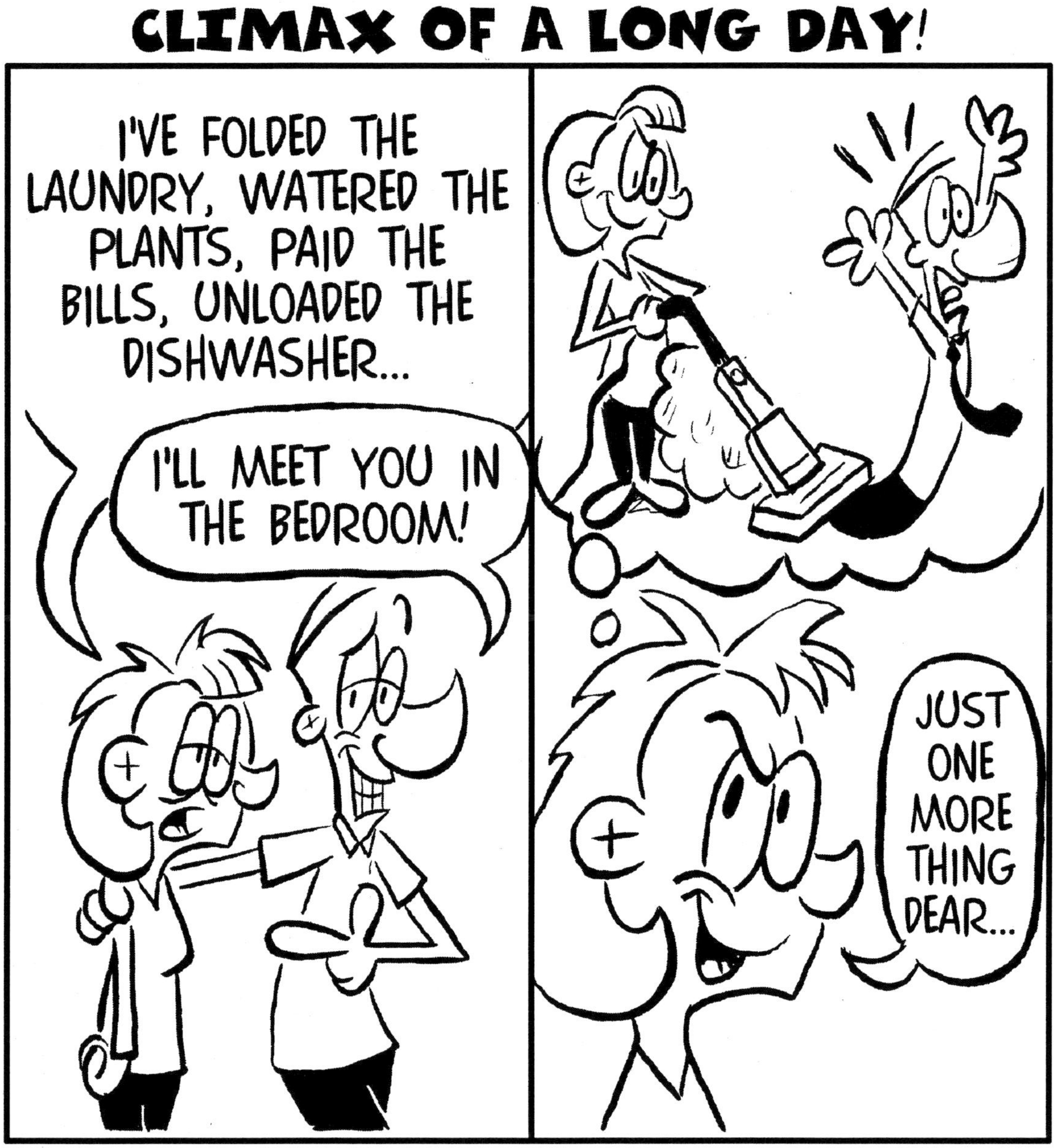
CLIMAX OF A LONG DAY!
I'VE FOLDED THE LAUNDRY, WATERED THE PLANTS, PAID THE BILLS, UNLOADED THE DISHWASHER...
I'LL MEET YOU IN THE BEDROOM!
JUST ONE MORE THING DEAR...

Women may feel overwhelmed during this period and less available to meet the needs of their family members.

CHARGED UP

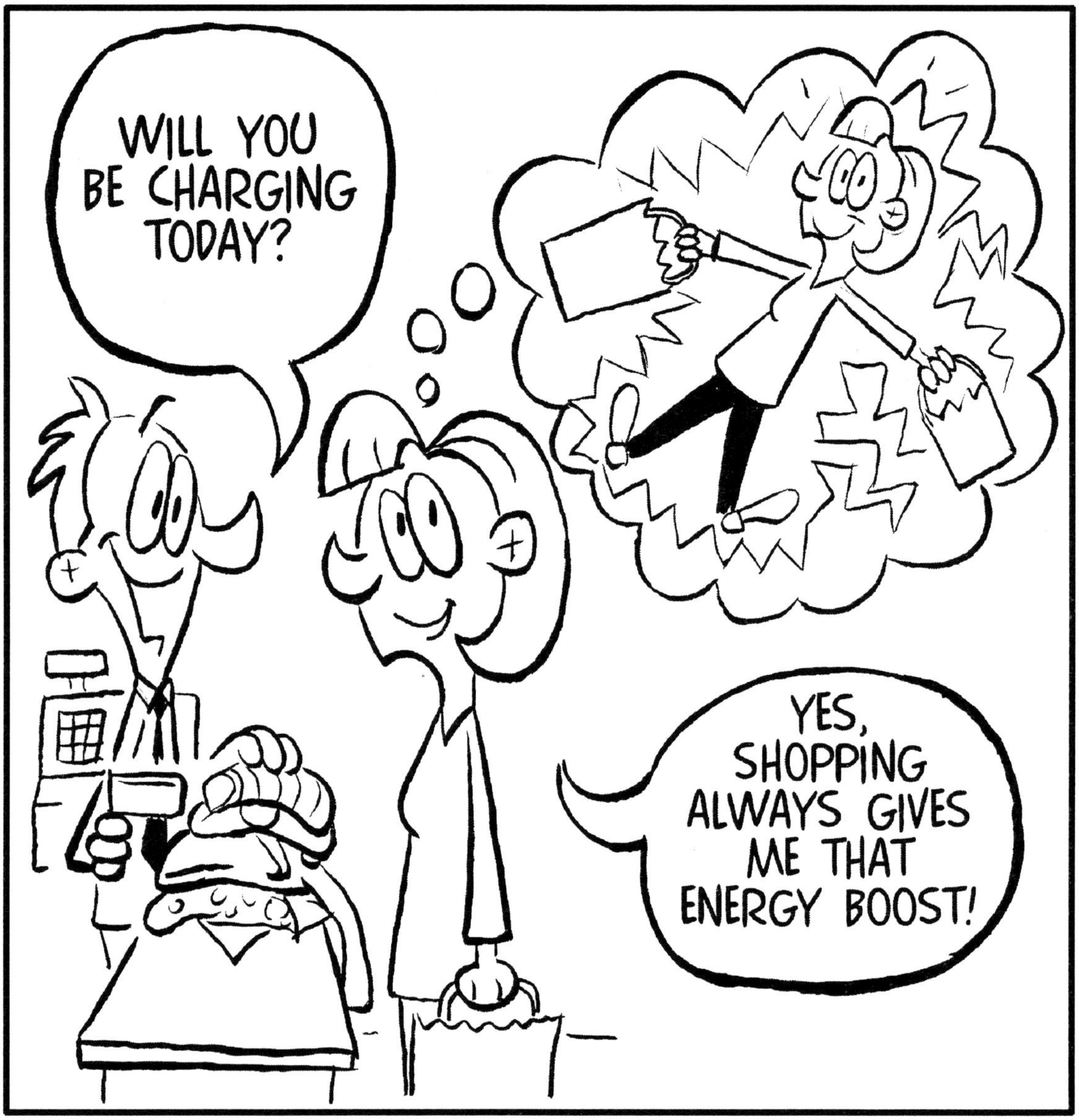
WILL YOU BE CHARGING TODAY?
YES, SHOPPING ALWAYS GIVES ME THAT ENERGY BOOST!

Many women consider supplemental vitamins, natural herbs, enzymes, or other ways to regain diminished energy. Maintain a balanced, nutritious diet. Consider eating more fresh, unprocessed food, at least five daily servings of fruits and vegetables, plenty of fiber, two daily servings of lean protein, and foods containing omega -3 fats.

Chapter Two

Marriage and Menopause

FOR BETTER OR WORSE

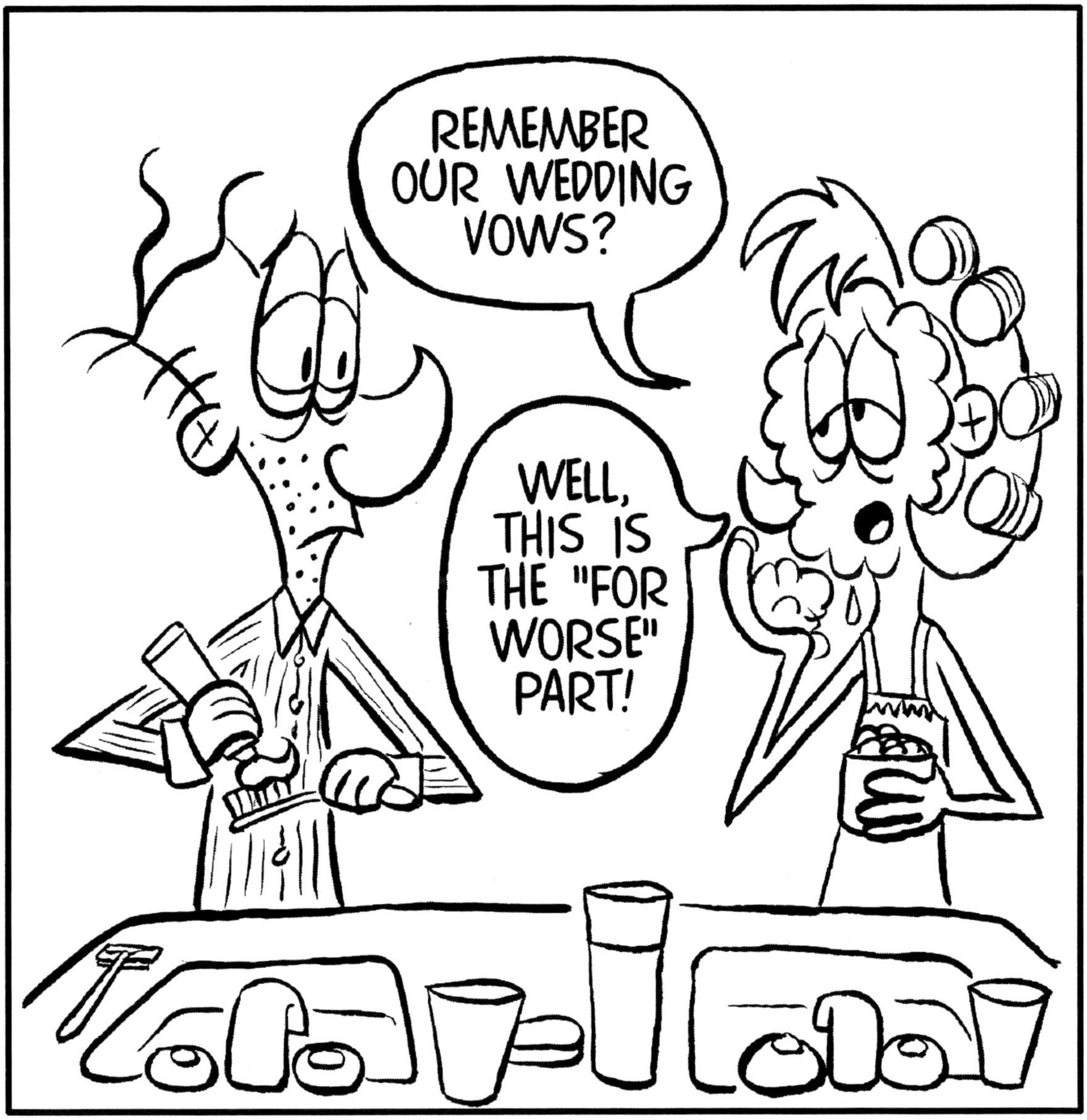
REMEMBER OUR WEDDING VOWS?
WELL, THIS IS THE "FOR WORSE" PART!

Marriages are often put to the test by increased conflict during this time.

WET DREAMS

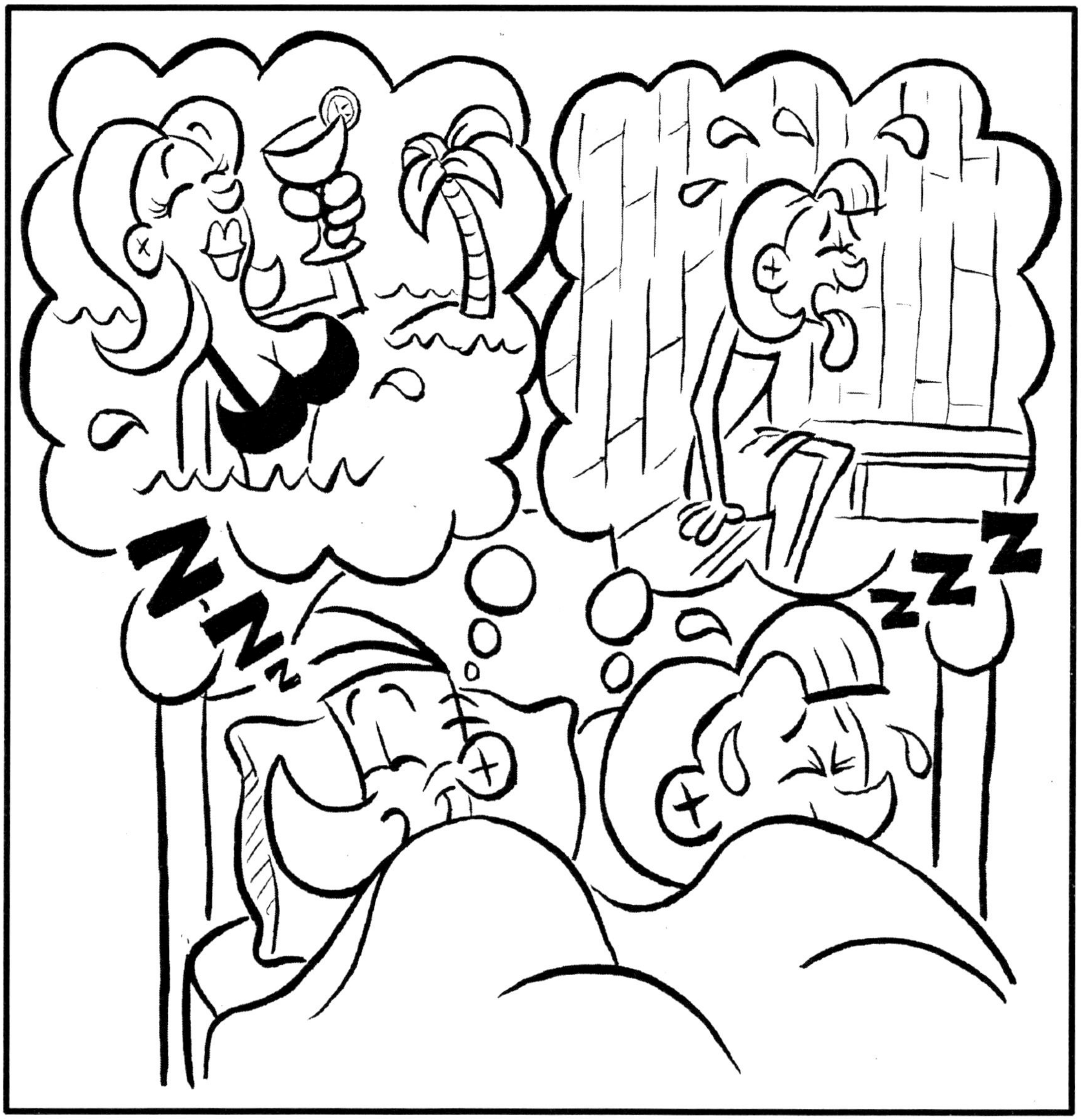

Clearly, your partner's mind may be in a very different place.

THE KISS

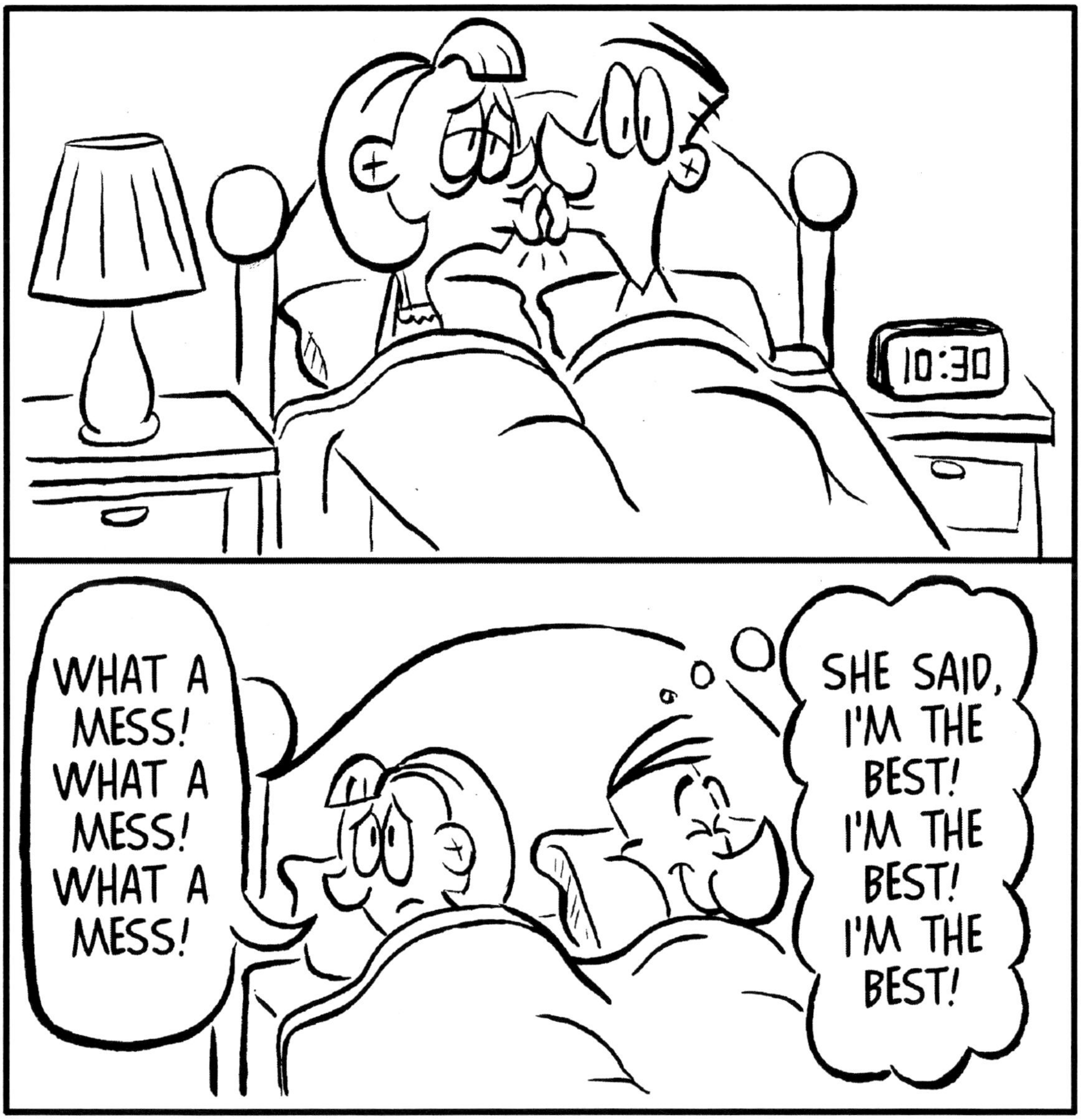
10:30
WHAT A MESS! WHAT A MESS! WHAT A MESS!
SHE SAID, I'M THE BEST! I'M THE BEST! I'M THE BEST!

Messages sent are not always messages received.

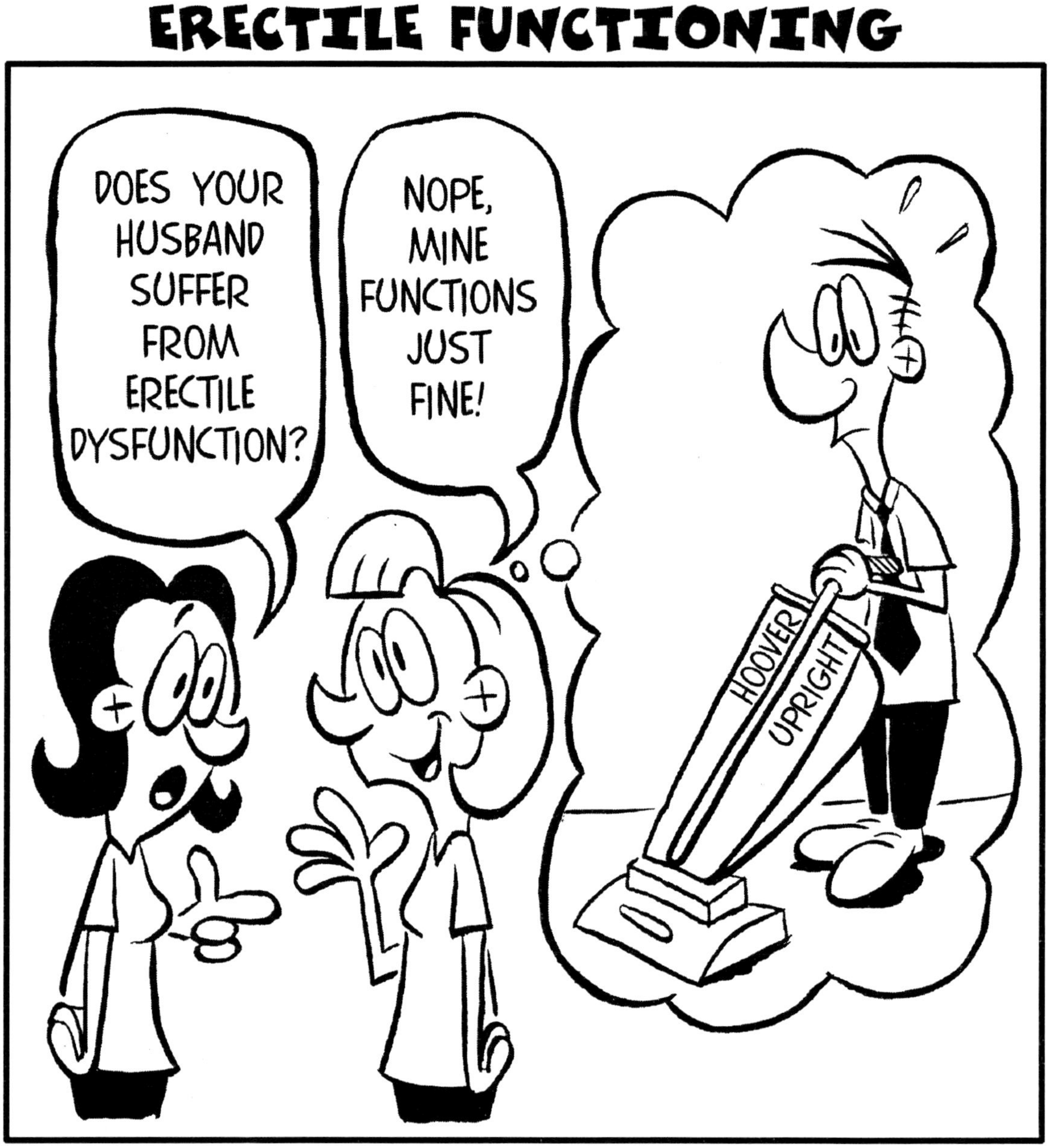
ERECTILE FUNCTIONING
DOES YOUR HUSBAND SUFFER FROM ERECTILE DYSFUNCTION?
NOPE, MINE FUNCTIONS JUST FINE!
HOOVER
UPRIGHT

Women are generally very appreciative of their partner's increased willingness to help with household chores.

MENOPAUSE MARKETPLACE

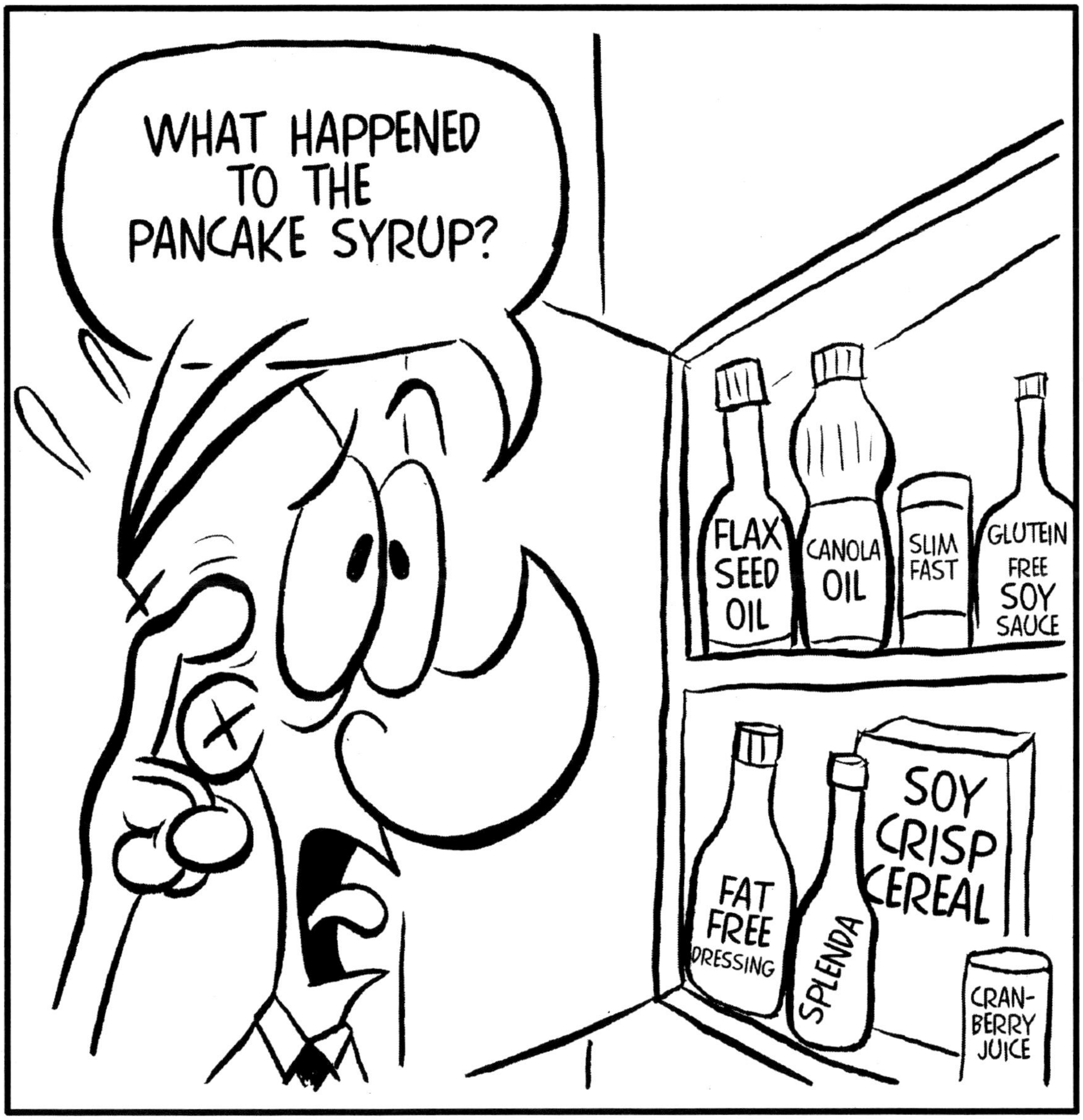

As women begin to explore healthy alternatives, family members may require some explanation about the changing composition of their refrigerators and pantries.

OUTER SPACE

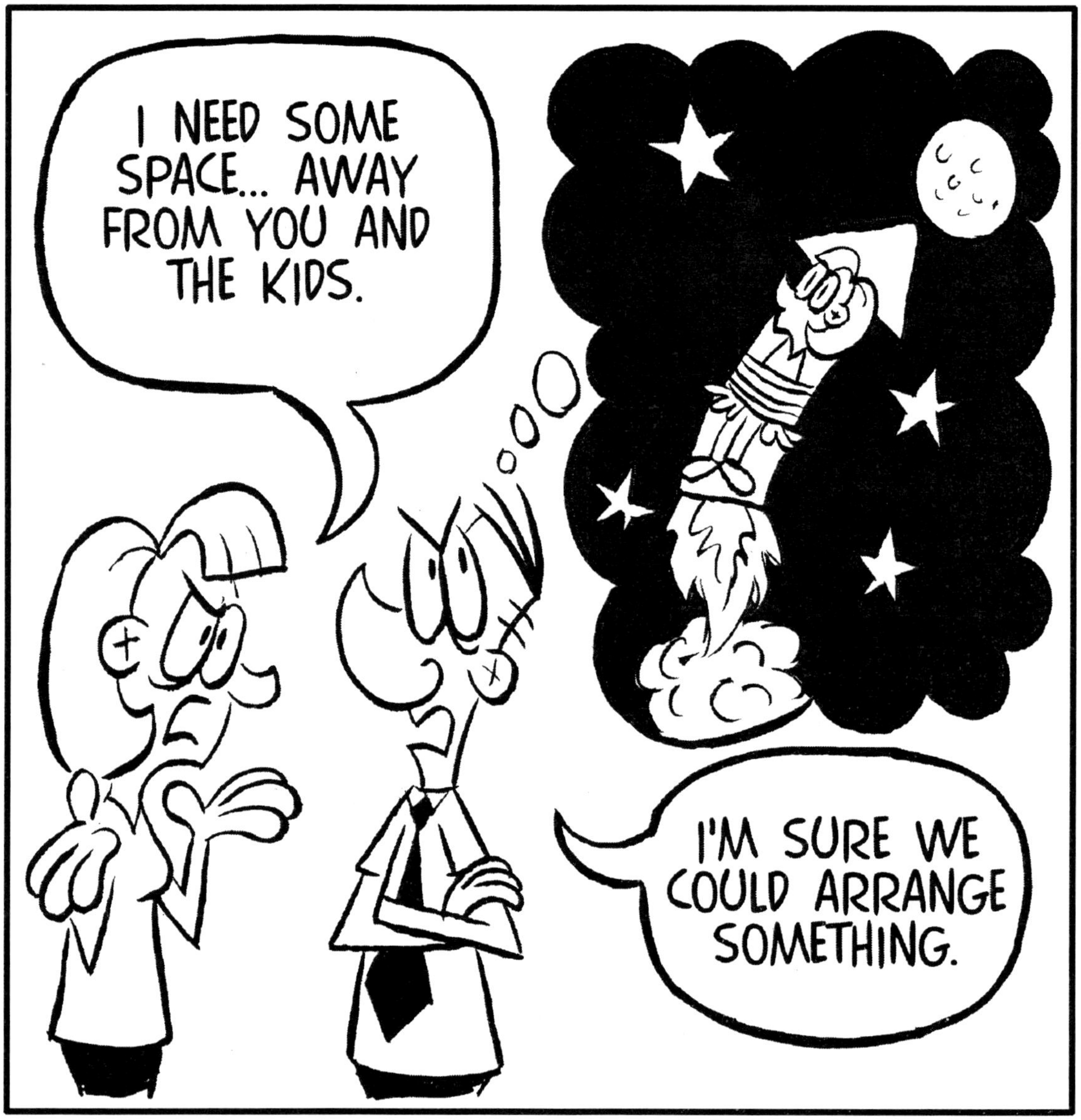
I NEED SOME SPACE... AWAY FROM YOU AND THE KIDS.
I'M SURE WE COULD ARRANGE SOMETHING.

During their menopausal years, women often express the need for more time alone. This may be associated with a traceable decrease in the brain chemical Oxytocin, often referred to as the "caretaking chemical."

FUTURE SHOCK

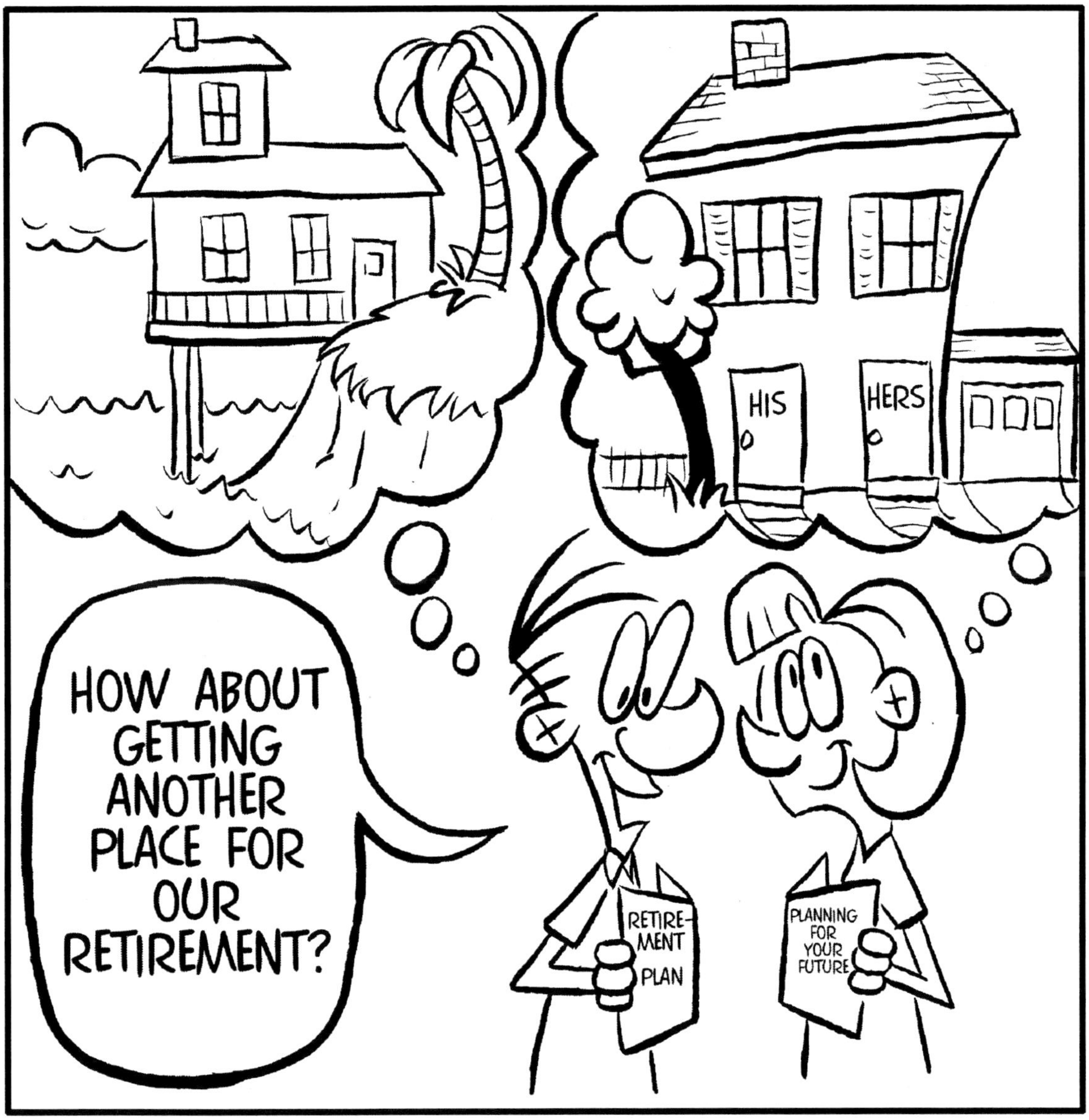
HIS
HERS
HOW ABOUT GETTING ANOTHER PLACE FOR OUR RETIREMENT?
RETIRE-MENT PLAN
PLANNING FOR YOUR FUTURE

As a consequence of the physical and mental changes caused by menopause, a significant number of divorces are initiated by women over the age of fifty.

Chapter Three

Motherhood and Menopause

KNOW IT ALL

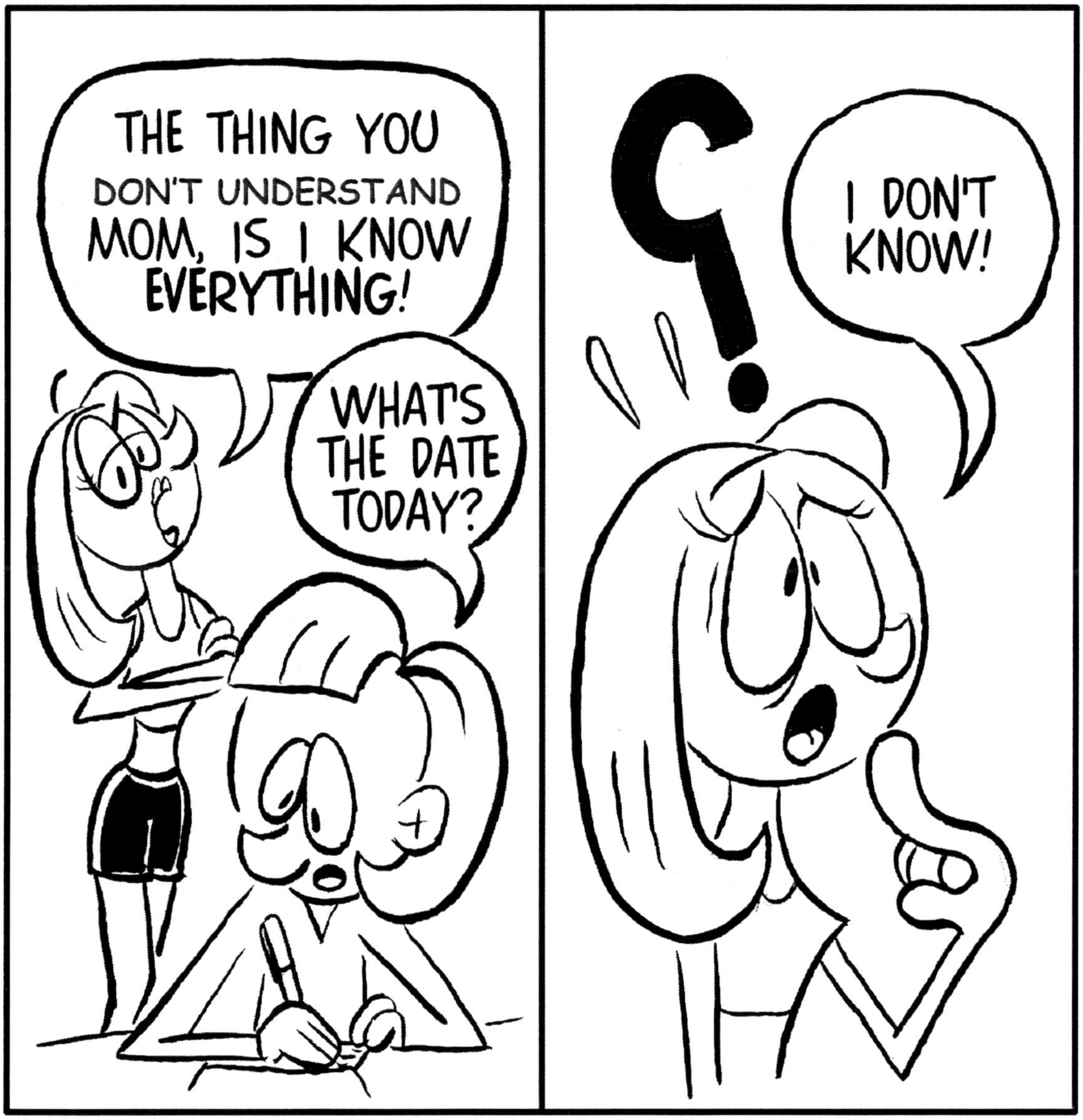
THE THING YOU DON'T UNDERSTAND MOM, IS I KNOW EVERYTHING!
WHAT'S THE DATE TODAY?
I DON'T KNOW!

Relationships with children, especially teen-aged children, may be challenging, for they too are experiencing great hormonal changes.

CLOSING THE GENERATION GAP

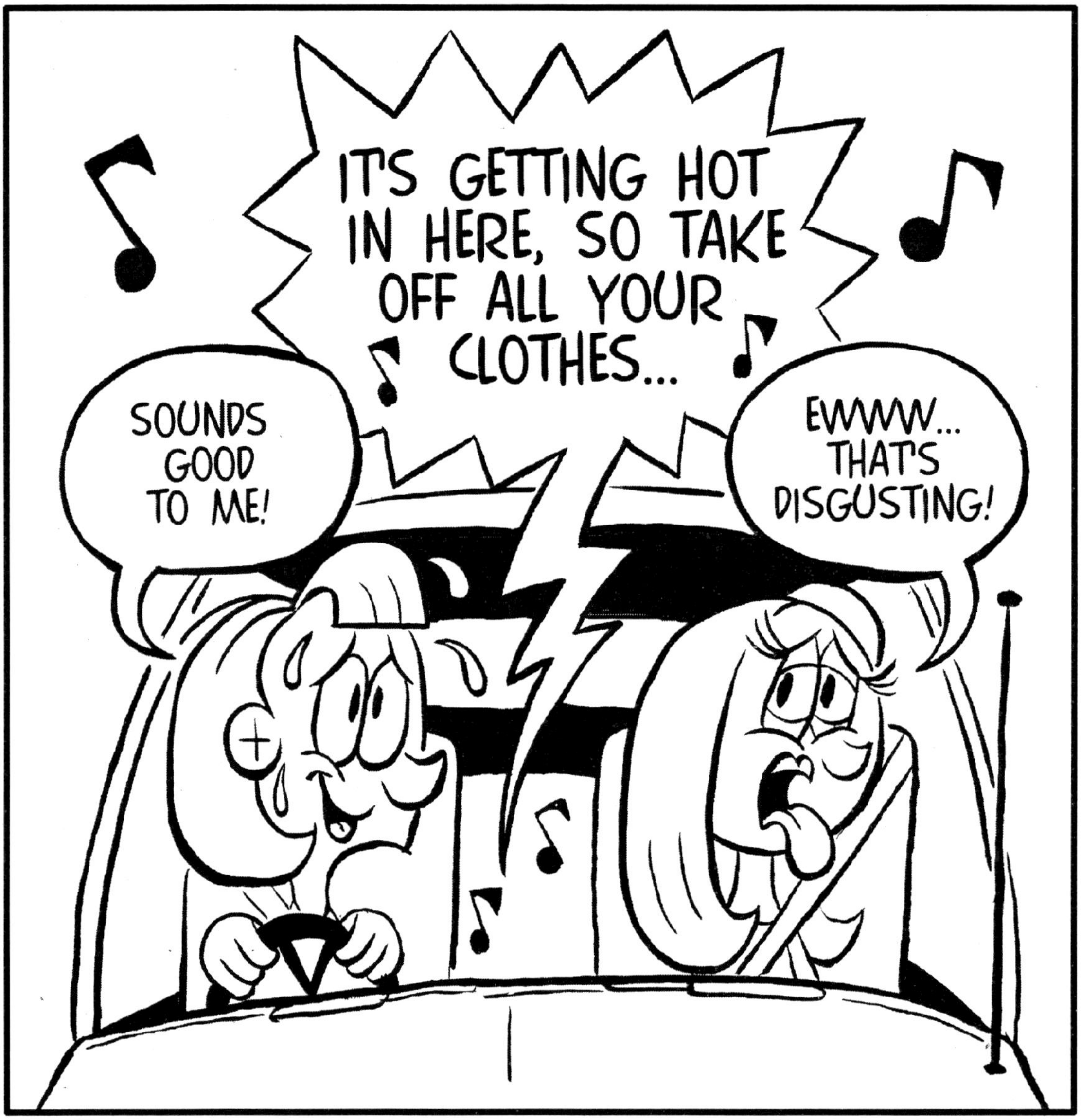
IT'S GETTING HOT IN HERE, SO TAKE OFF ALL YOUR CLOTHES...
SOUNDS GOOD TO ME!
EWWW... THAT'S DISGUSTING!

A mother's attempt to relate to her child may not always be appreciated. Still, a car ride is a good place to listen and share.

TEEN CUISINE

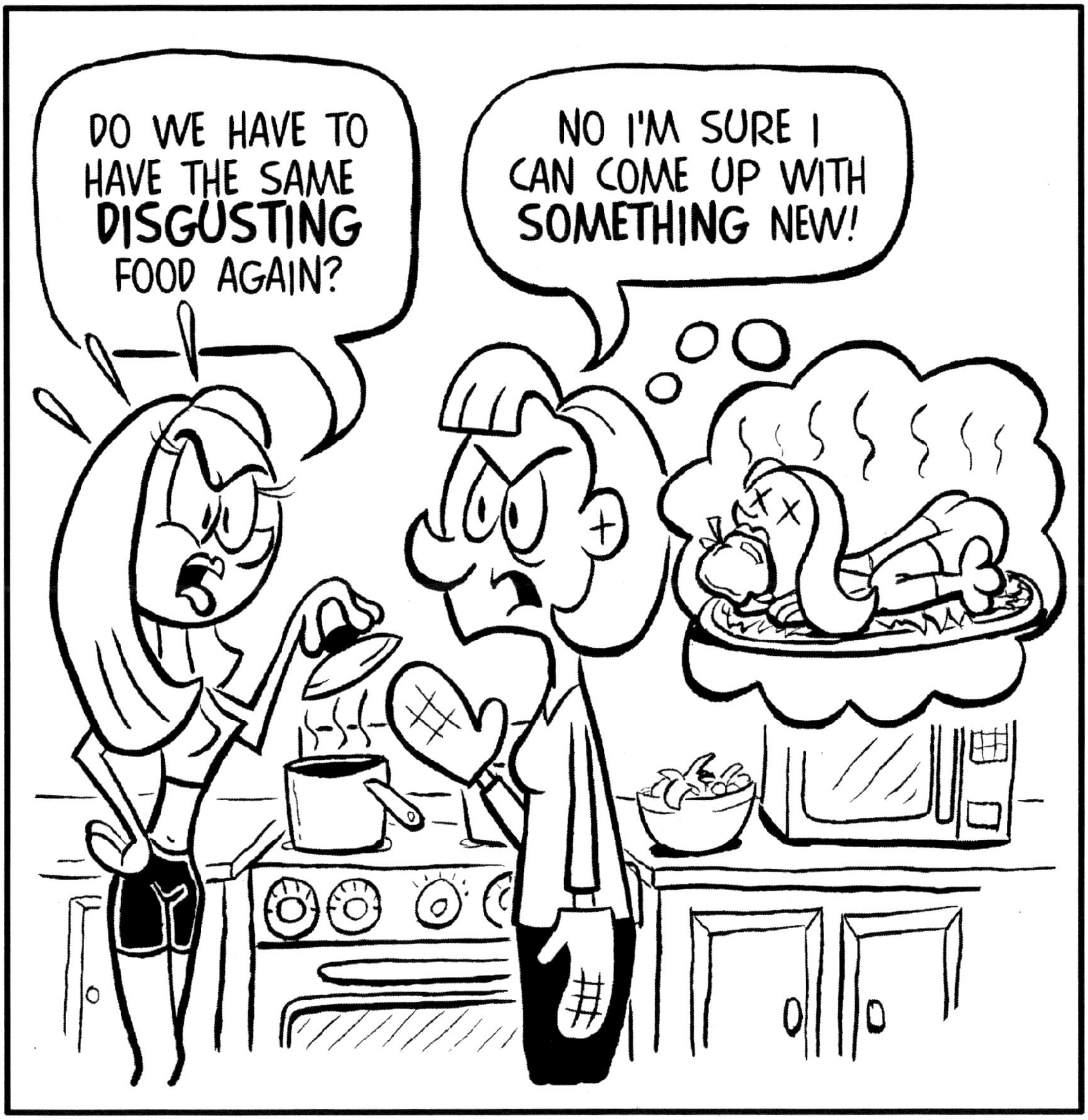
DO WE HAVE TO HAVE THE SAME DISGUSTING FOOD AGAIN?
NO I'M SURE I CAN COME UP WITH SOMETHING NEW!

Simple things that were once valued may now be considered unacceptable.

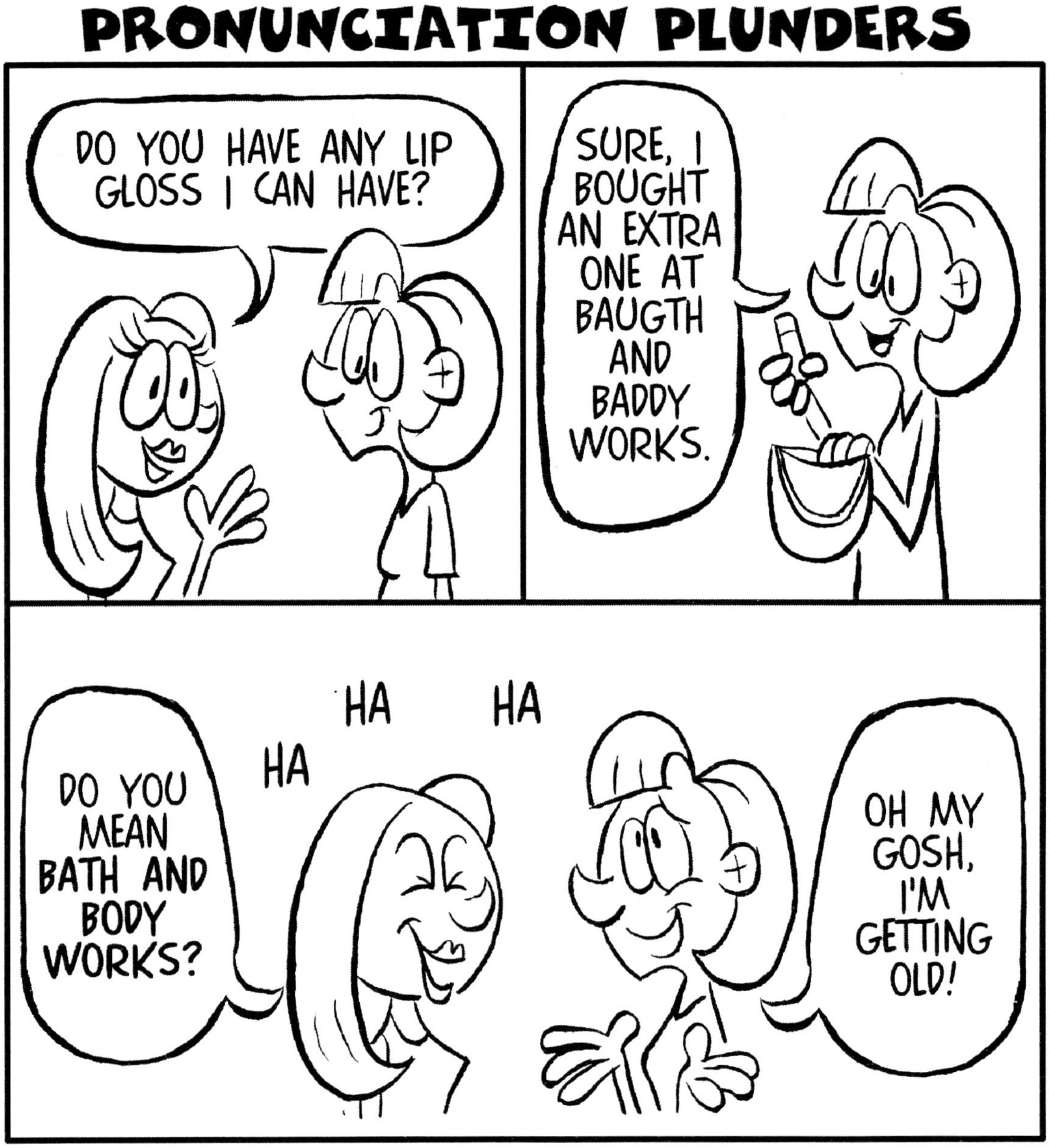
PRONUNCIATION PLUNDERS
DO YOU HAVE ANY LIP GLOSS I CAN HAVE?
SURE, I BOUGHT AN EXTRA ONE AT BAUGTH AND BADDY WORKS.
DO YOU MEAN BATH AND BODY WORKS?
HA
HA
HA
OH MY GOSH, I'M GETTING OLD!

Slips of the tongue may become more frequent.

TEEN SCENE INVESTIGATIONS (TSI)

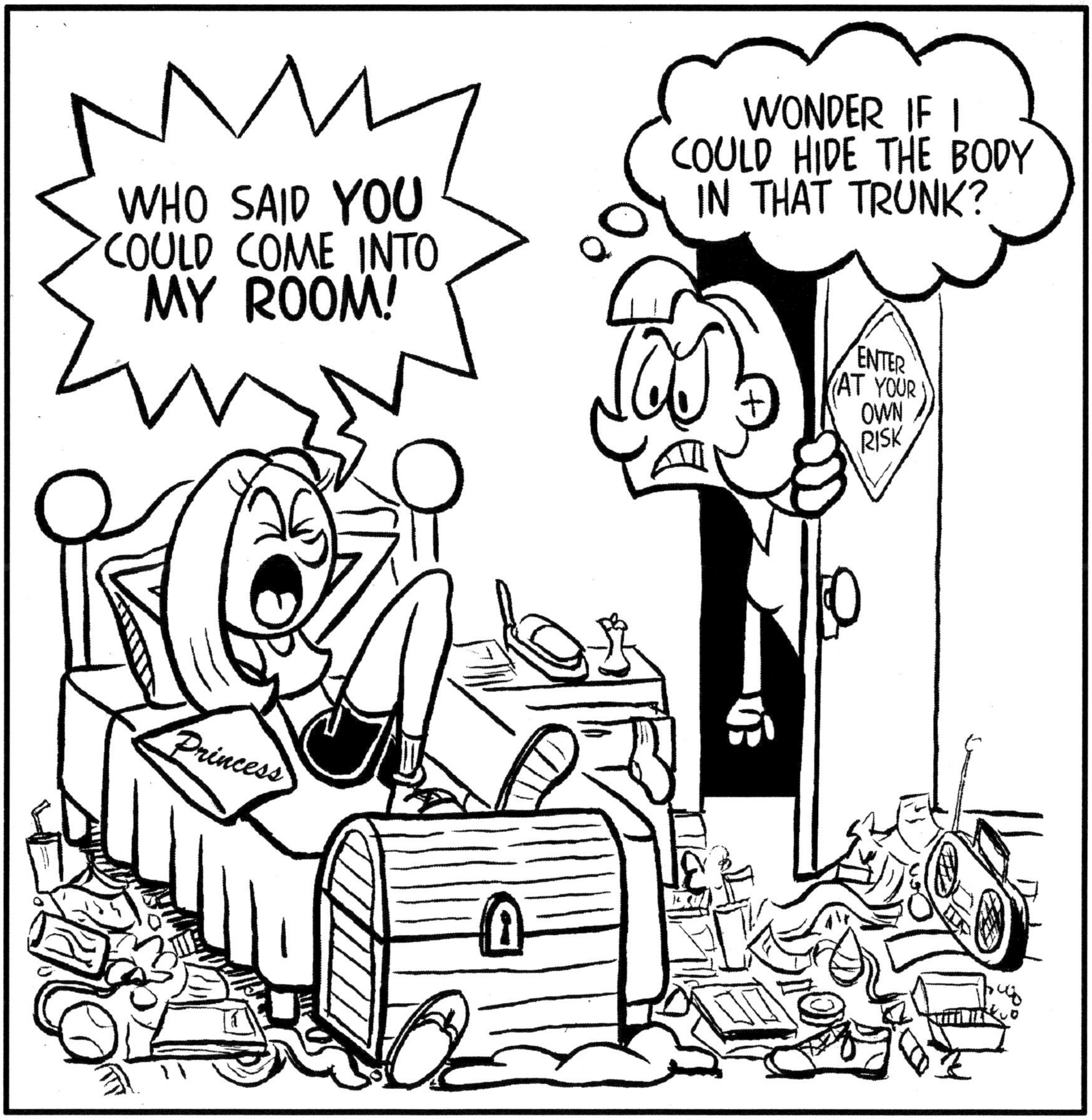
WHO SAID YOU COULD COME INTO MY ROOM!
WONDER IF I COULD HIDE THE BODY IN THAT TRUNK?
ENTER AT YOUR OWN RISK
Princess

The range of tolerance will be greatly tested during this period.

HERE'S LOOKIN' AT YA!

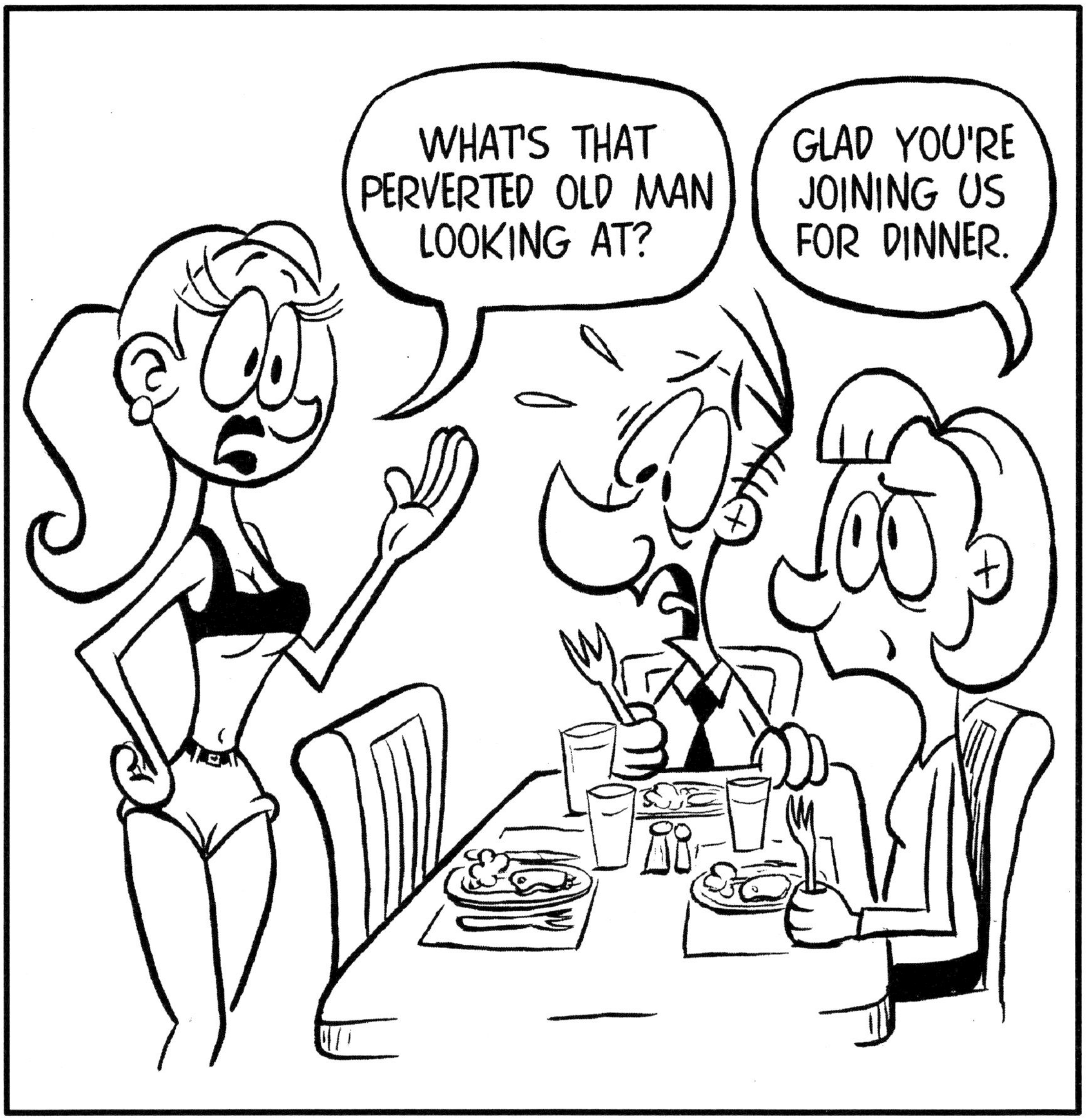
WHAT'S THAT PERVERTED OLD MAN LOOKING AT?
GLAD YOU'RE JOINING US FOR DINNER.

Family interactions may take on a new tone.

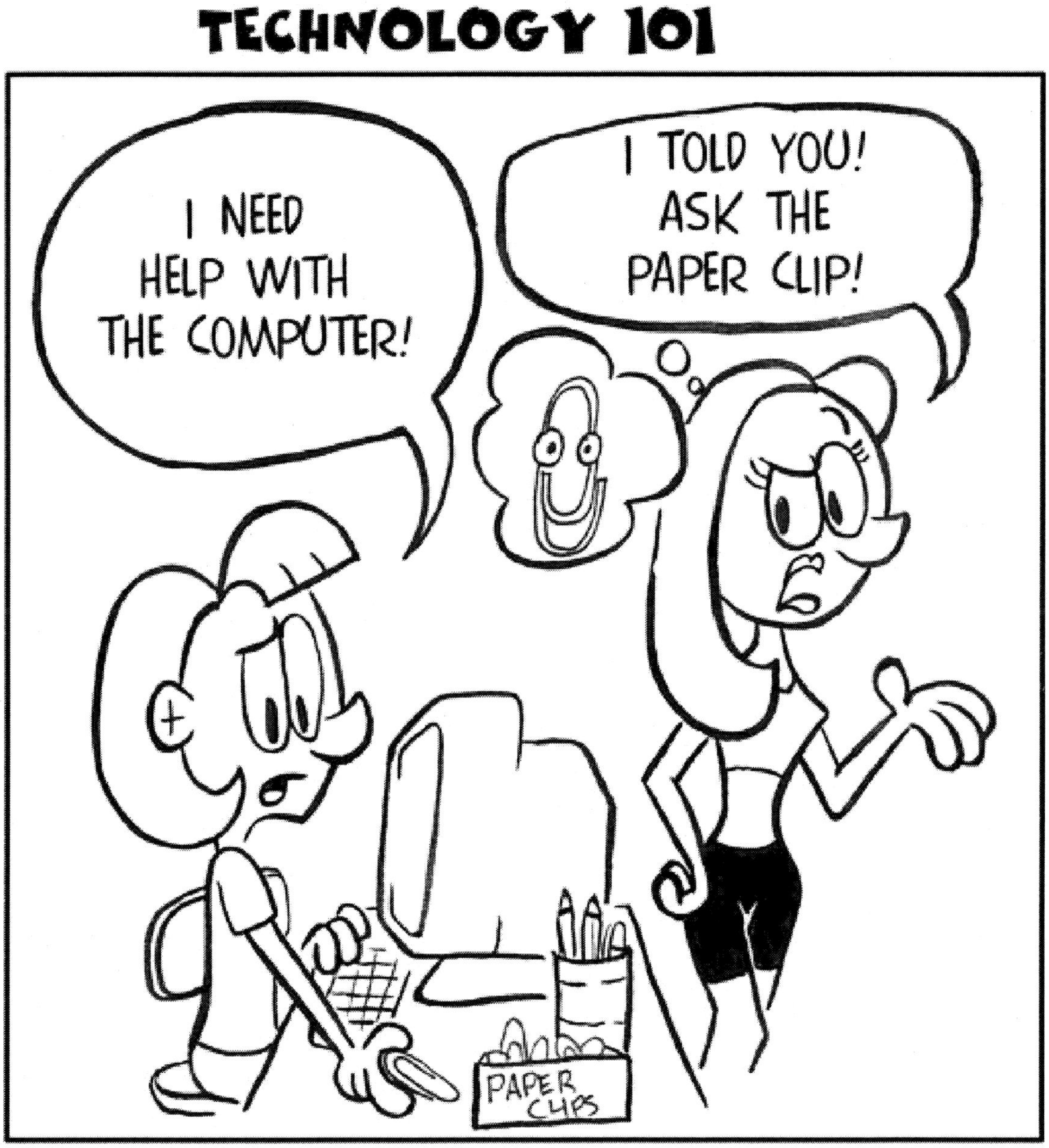
TECHNOLOGY 101
I NEED HELP WITH THE COMPUTER!
I TOLD YOU! ASK THE PAPER CLIP!
PAPER CLIPS

Familiar objects may take on new meanings.

HOMEWORK HAVEN

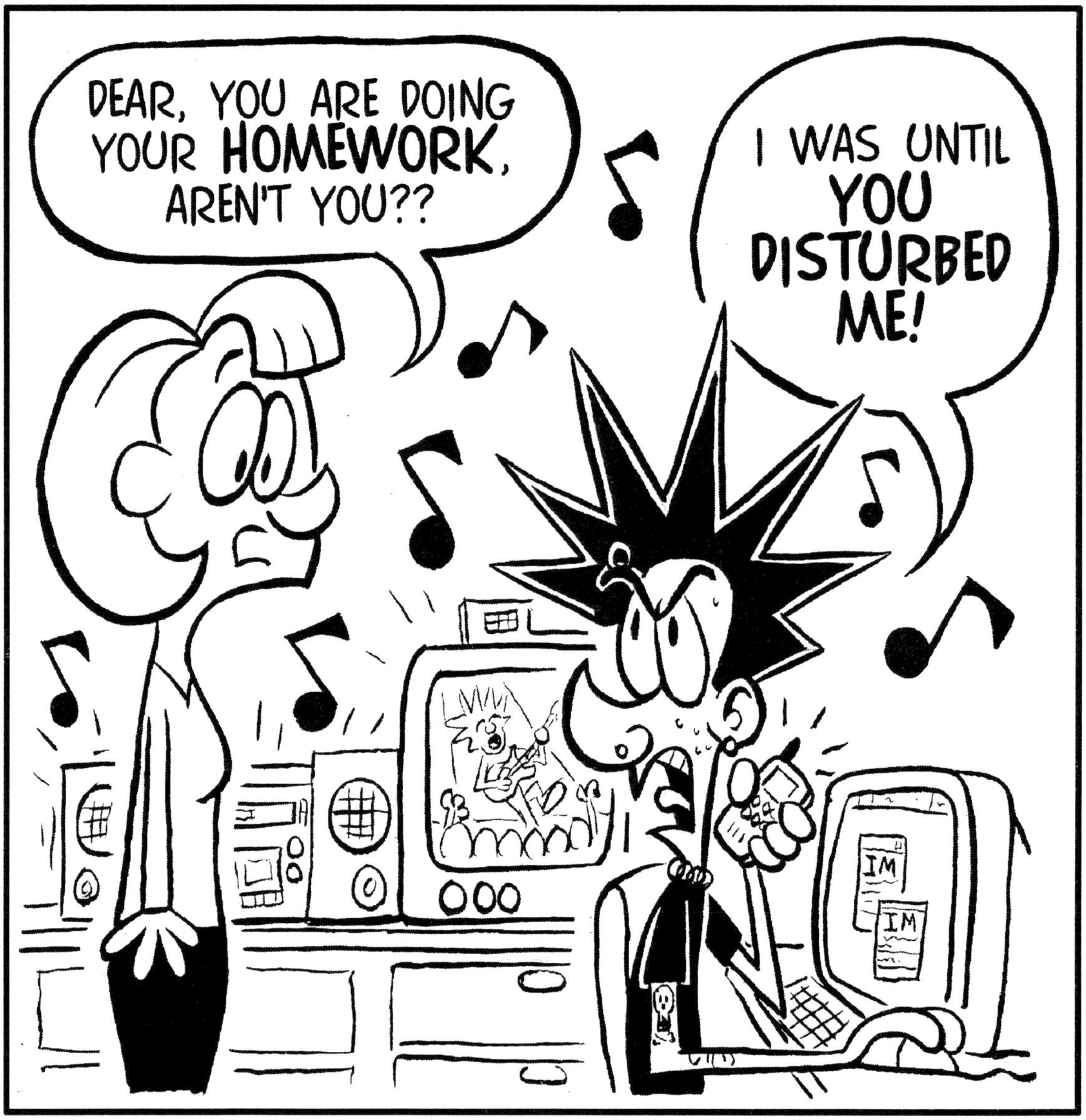
DEAR, YOU ARE DOING YOUR HOMEWORK, AREN'T YOU??
I WAS UNTIL YOU DISTURBED ME!
IM
IM

A mother's careful watch may no longer be appreciated.

Chapter Four

Generational Differences

A TIME OF LOSS

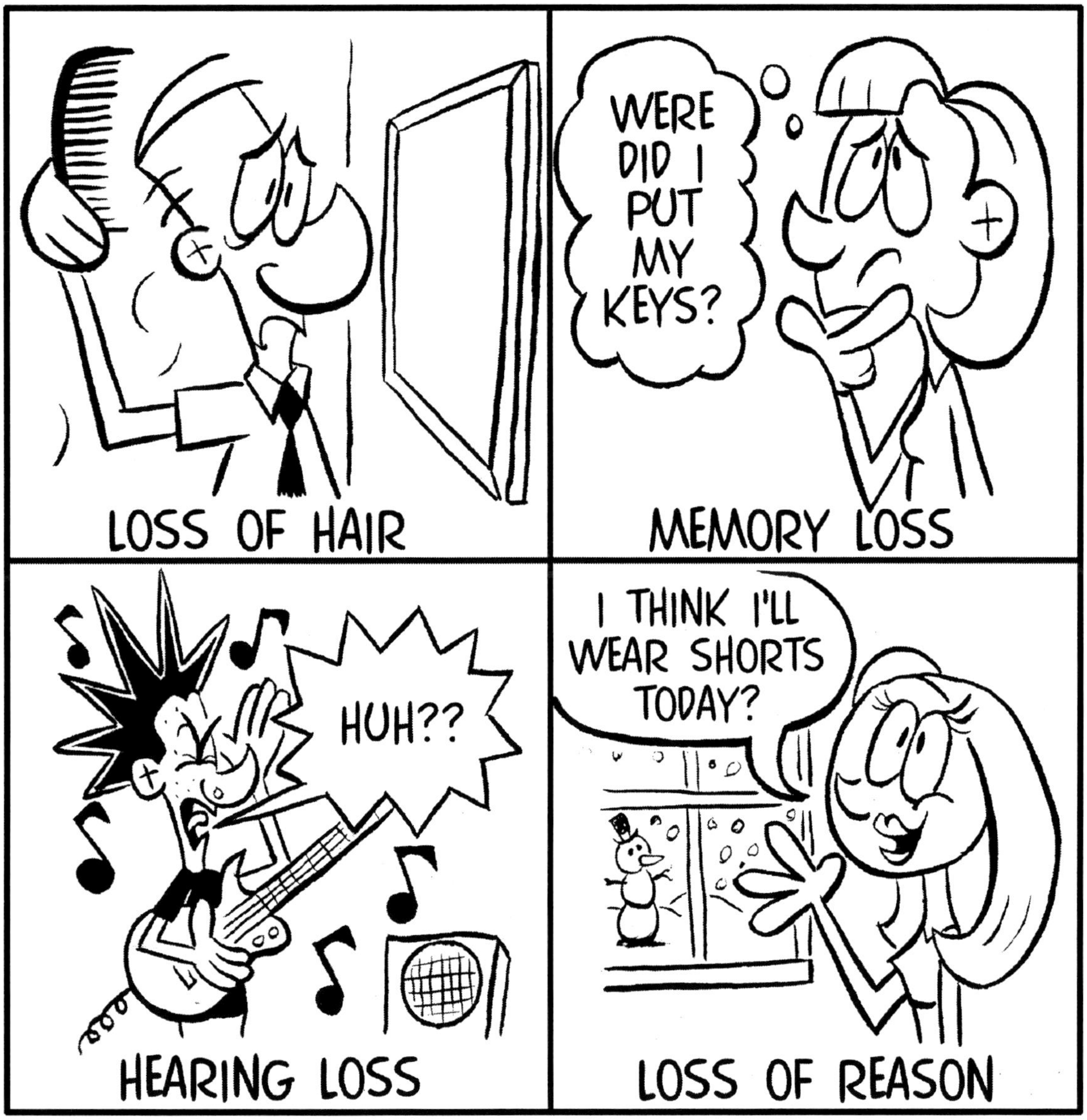
LOSS OF HAIR
WERE DID I PUT MY KEYS?
MEMORY LOSS
HUH??
HEARING LOSS
I THINK I'LL WEAR SHORTS TODAY?
LOSS OF REASON

Generational differences will become more apparent.

MEDITATIONS

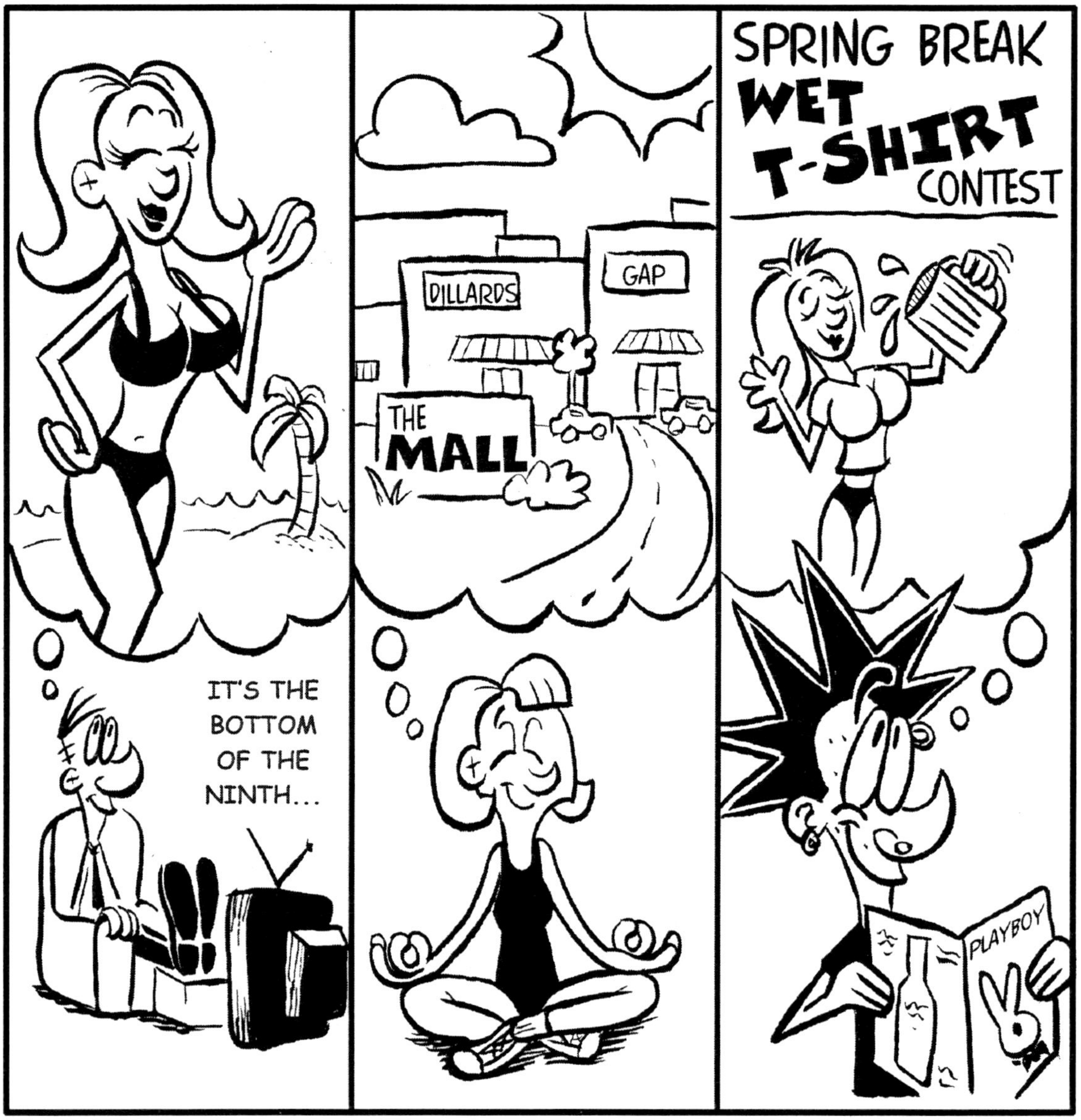

Daydreams among family members will become increasingly divergent and more personal in nature.

THE HEAT IS ON

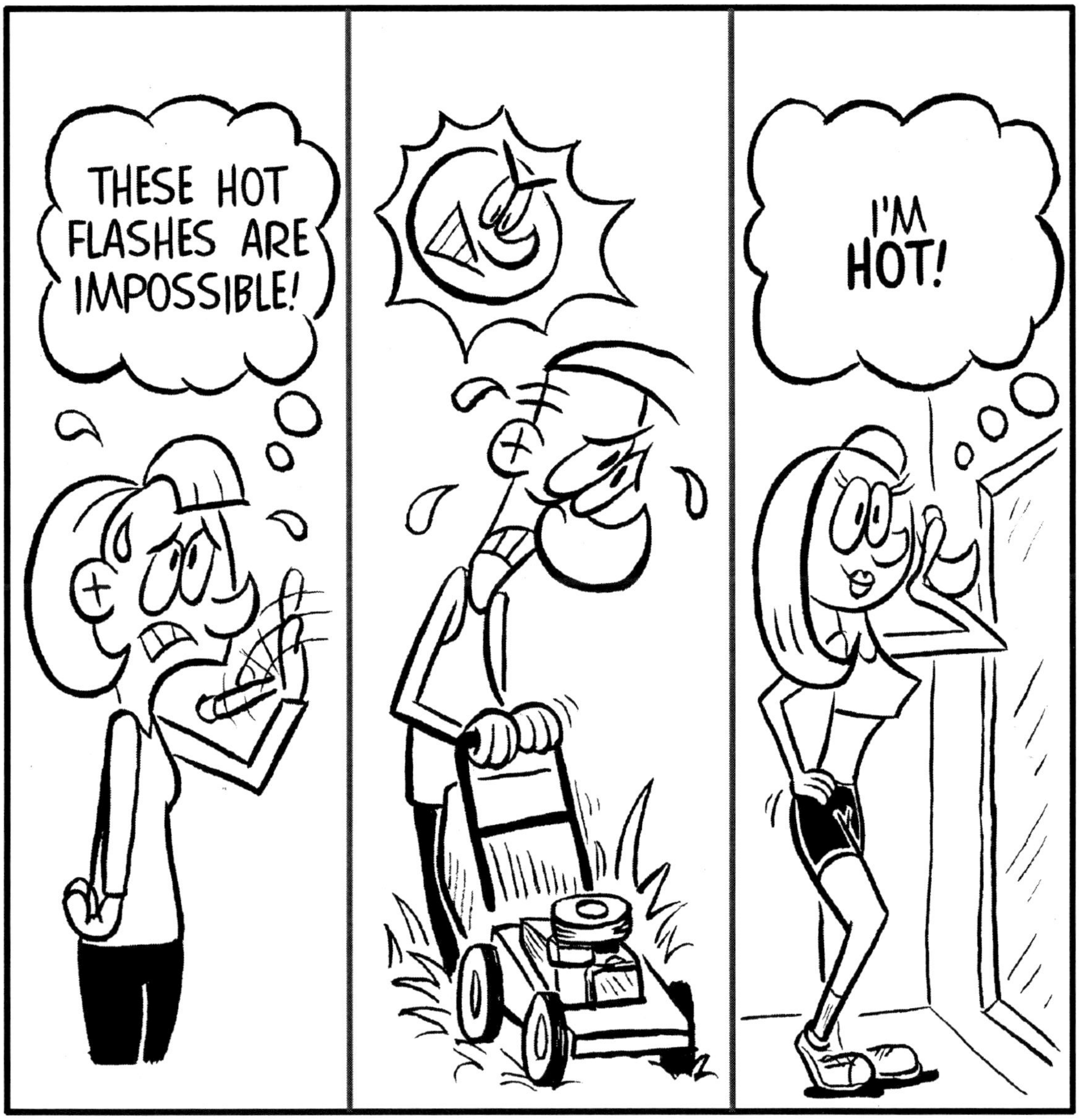

Once commonly understood expressions may begin to take on new meanings.

ON THE BALL

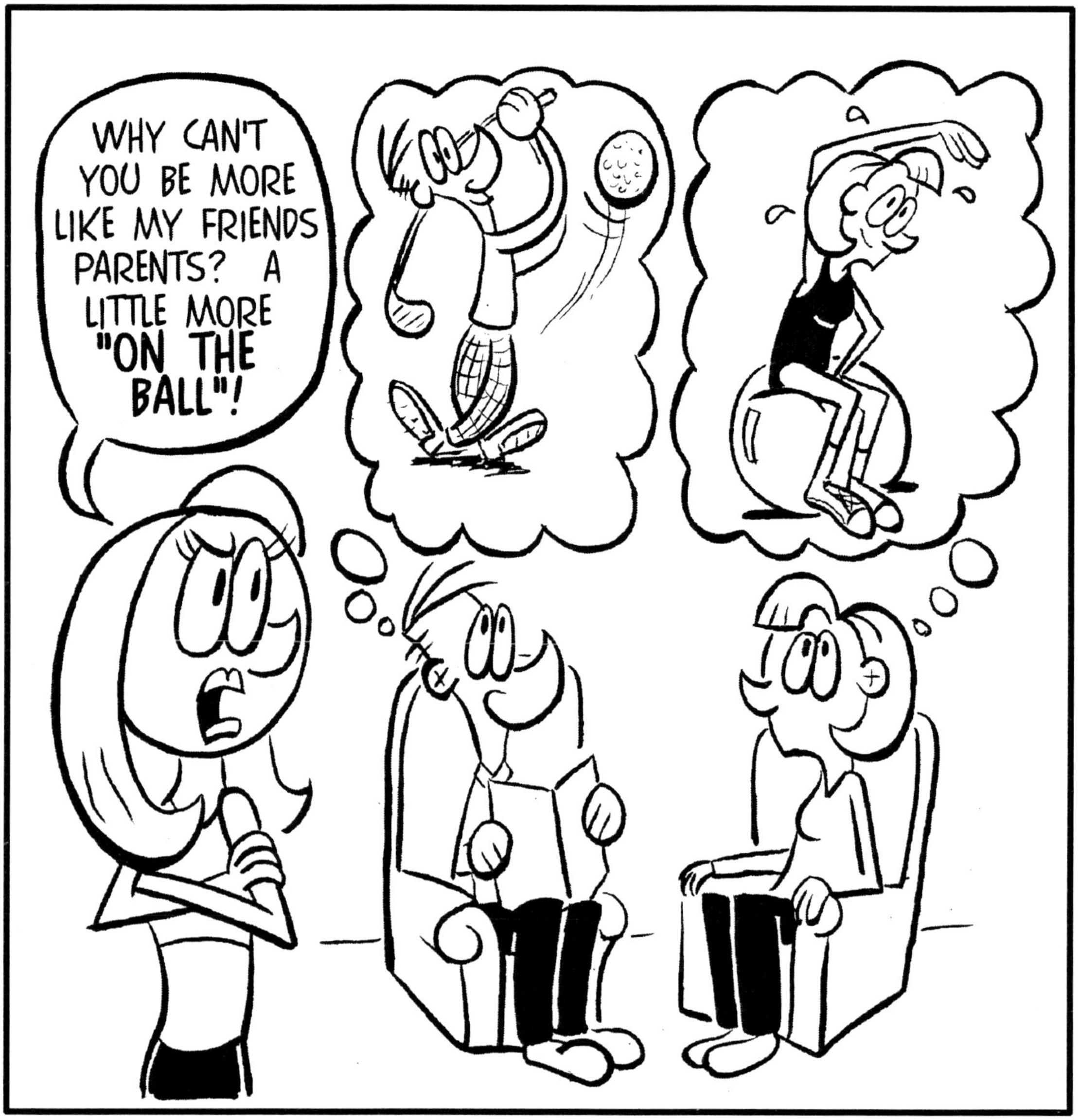
WHY CAN'T YOU BE MORE LIKE MY FRIENDS PARENTS? A LITTLE MORE "ON THE BALL"!

Mothers will find themselves contemplating amusing ways to thwart verbal attacks.

THE BIG LIFT

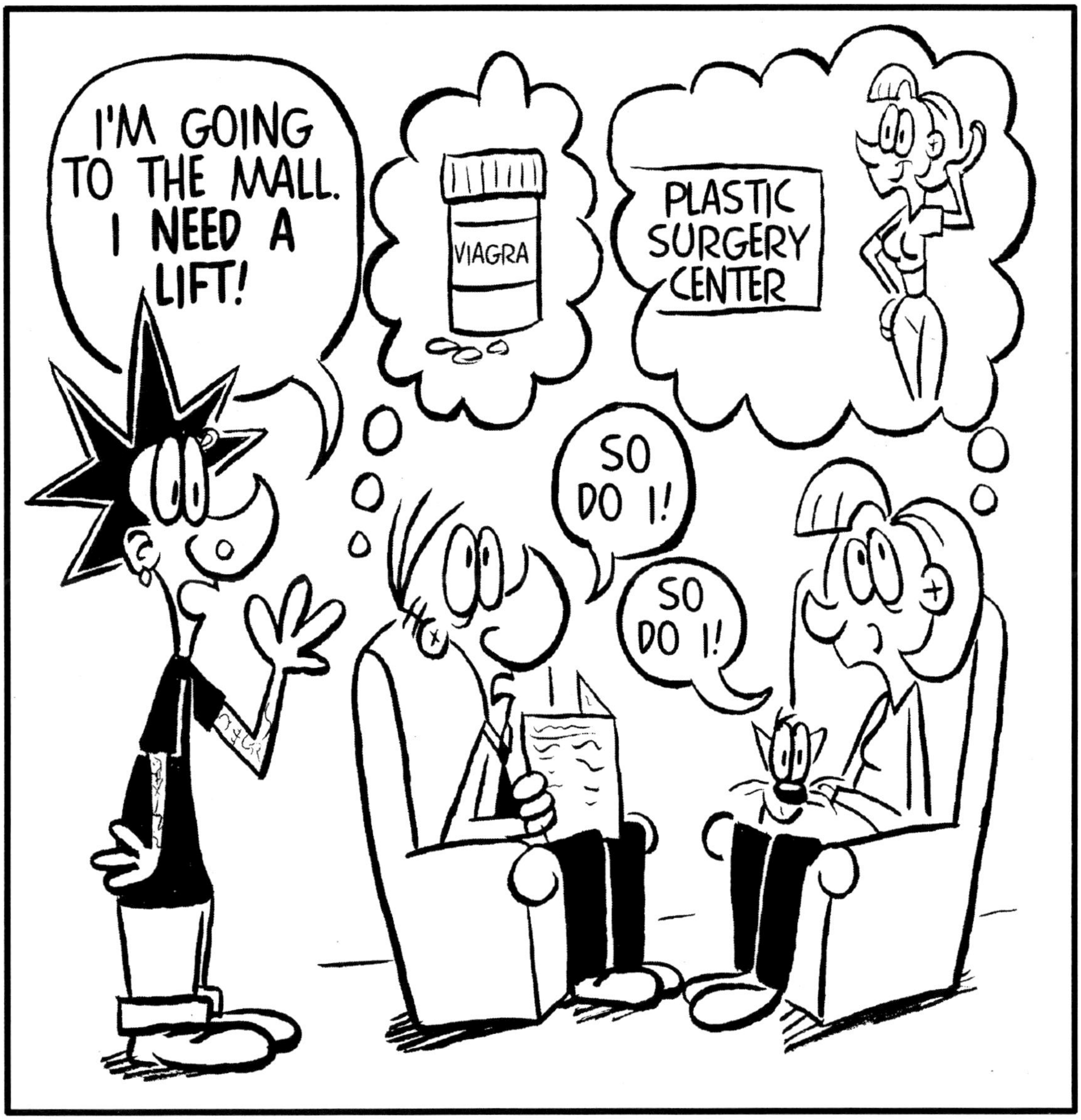
I'M GOING TO THE MALL. I NEED A LIFT!
VIAGRA
PLASTIC SURGERY CENTER
SO DO I!
SO DO I!

Simple requests may now take a few moments to sink in.

ENCOUNTERS OF A DIFFERENT NATURE

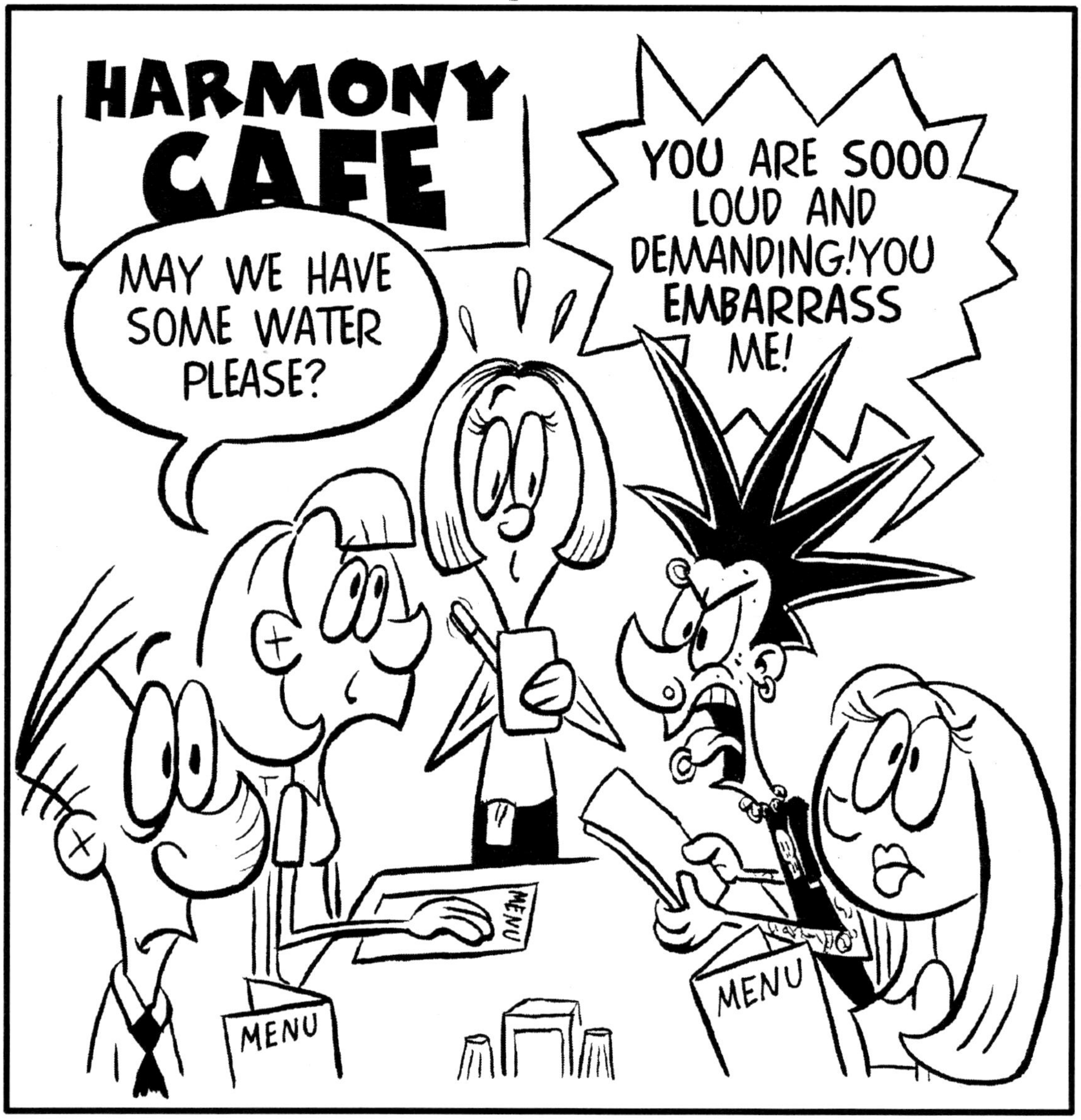
HARMONY CAFE
MAY WE HAVE SOME WATER PLEASE?
YOU ARE SOOO LOUD AND DEMANDING! YOU EMBARRASS ME!
MENU
MENU
MENU

Your once typical behaviors may suddenly become a source of irritation or embarrassment.

THE ULTIMATE POWER

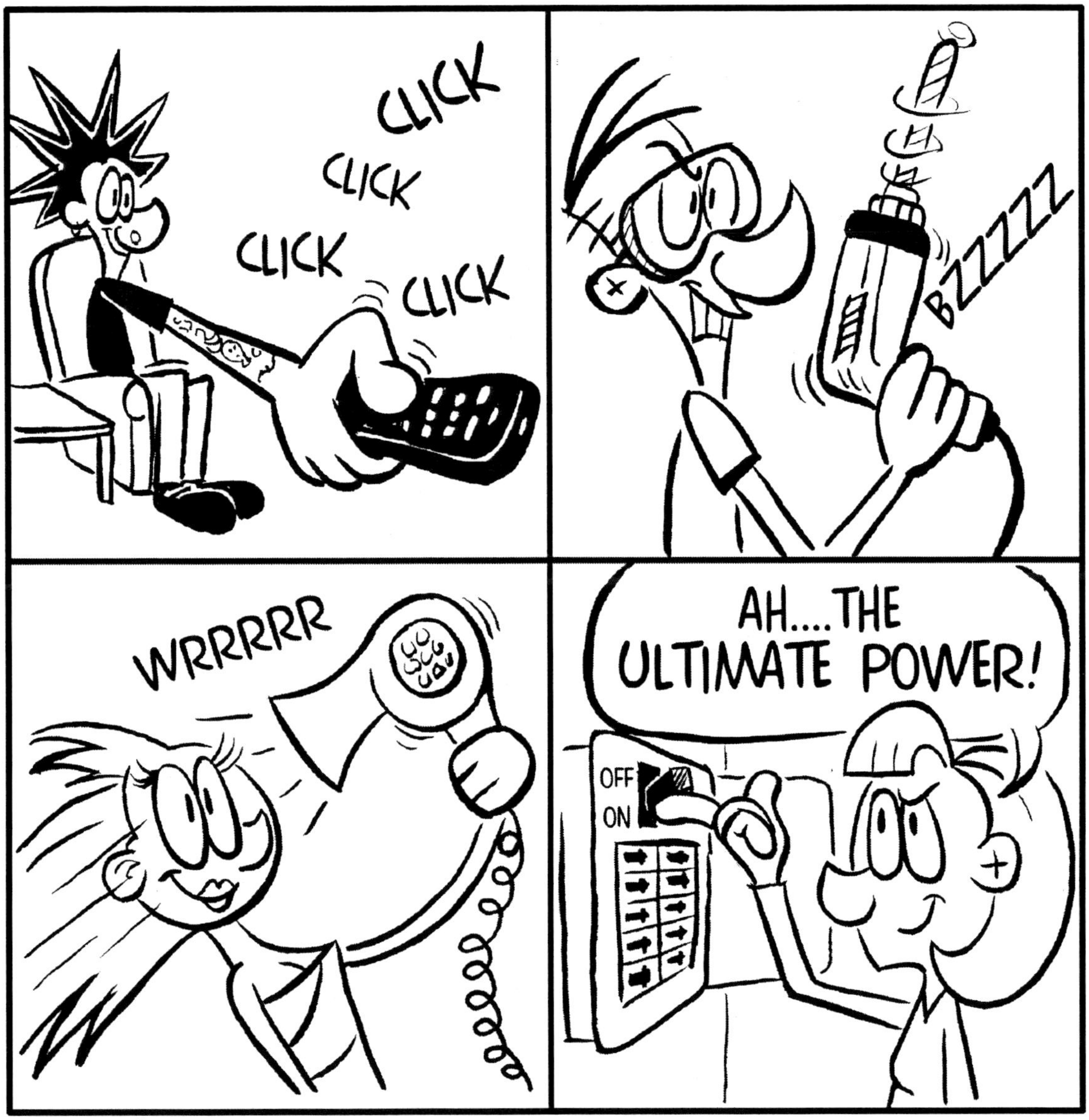

Remember that if tested, women can become extremely resilient and very powerful.

Chapter Five

Preventative Maintenance

PAIN IN THE NECK

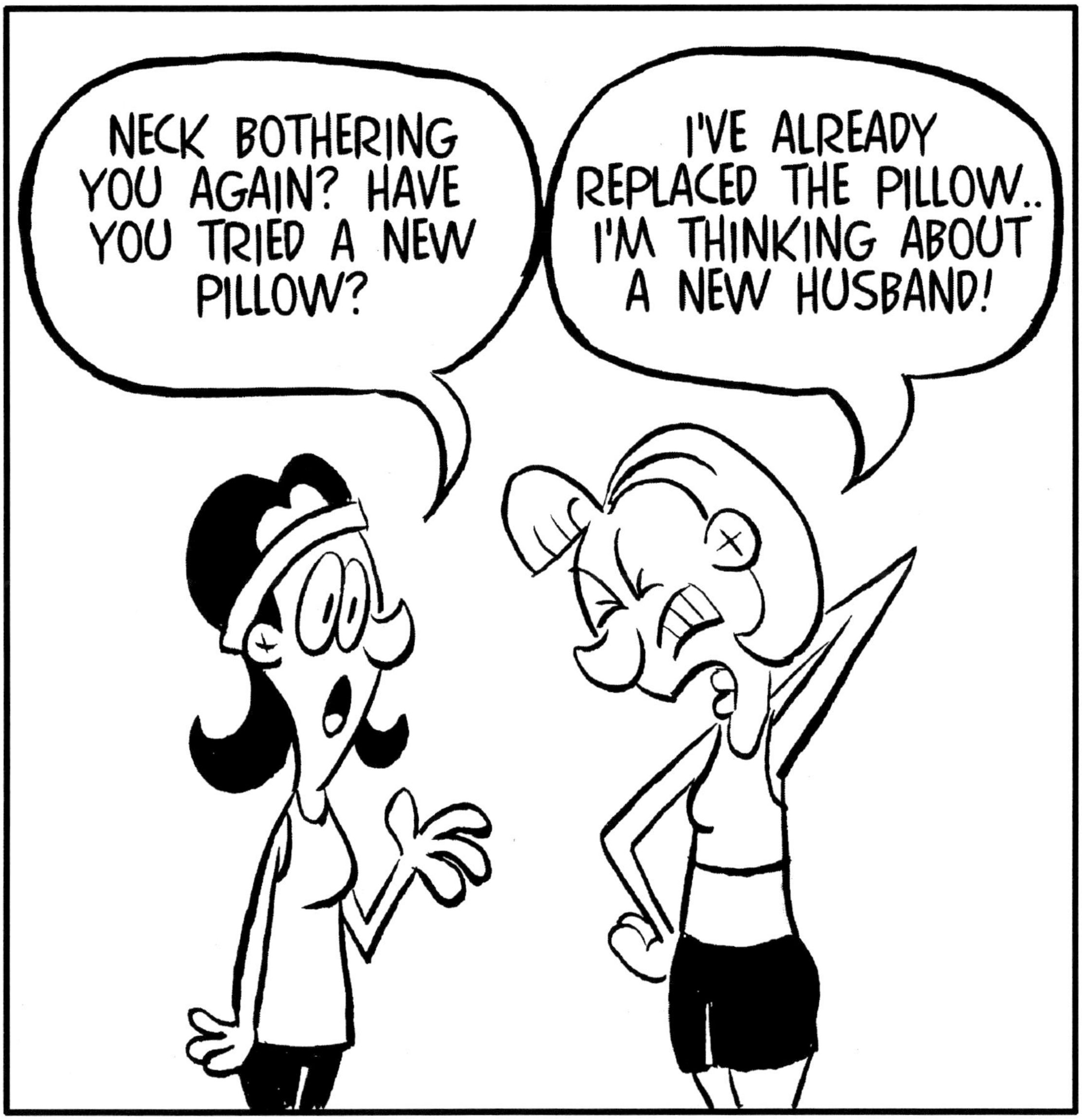
NECK BOTHERING YOU AGAIN? HAVE YOU TRIED A NEW PILLOW?
I'VE ALREADY REPLACED THE PILLOW.. I'M THINKING ABOUT A NEW HUSBAND!

Increased aches and pains, primarily in the neck, wrist, hips, or spine, may be signs that bone mineral density is changing. Calcium with Vitamin D and Magnesium supplements are recommended. Glucosamine and Methylsulfonylmethane (MSM), are natural supplements that are widely used to rebuild cartilage and relieve inflammation, respectively. Consider a bone density scan every two years from the onset of menopause, or sooner, depending on symptoms or family history.

HRT HOTLINE

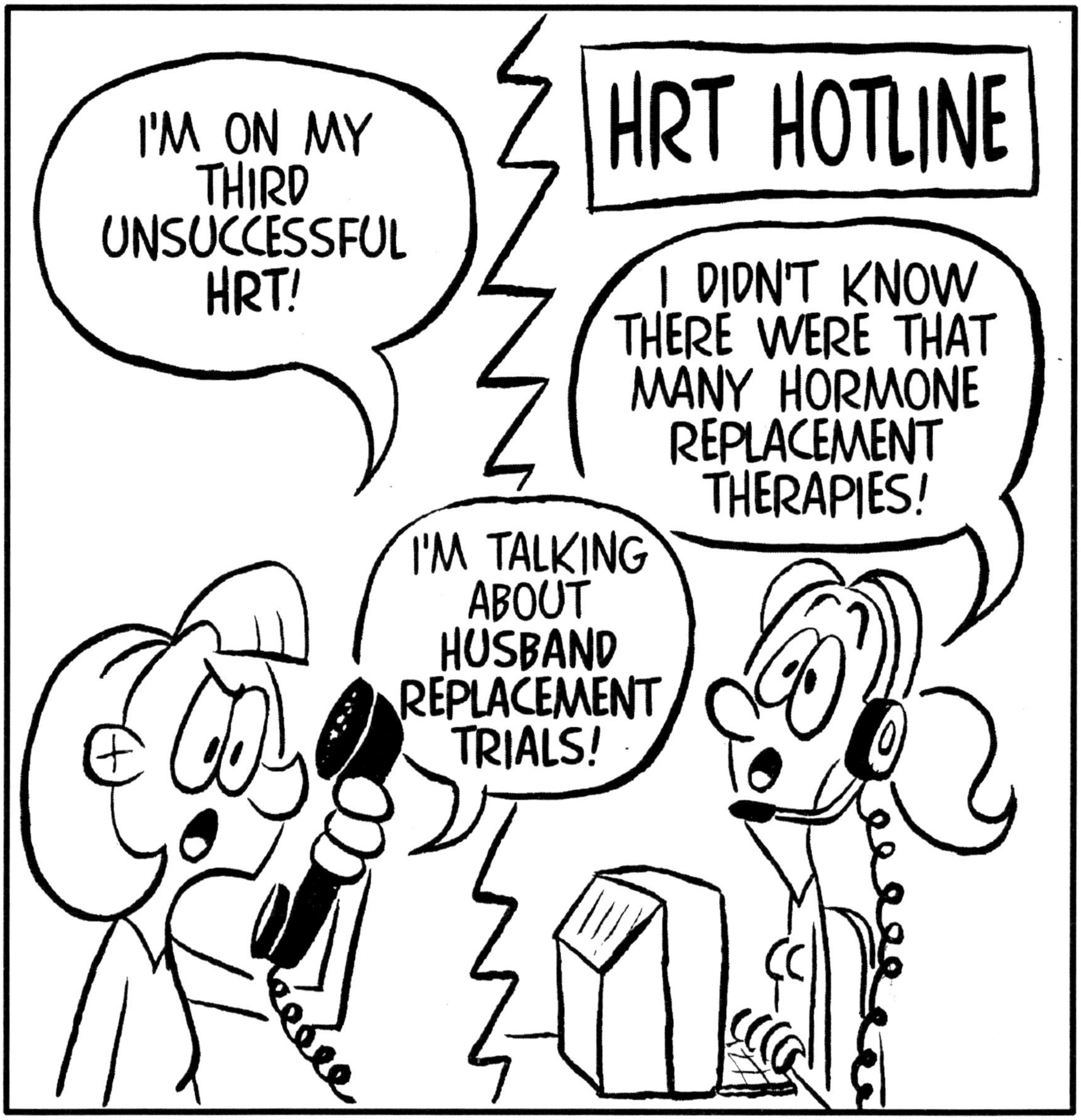
HRT HOTLINE
I'M ON MY THIRD UNSUCCESSFUL HRT!
I DIDN'T KNOW THERE WERE THAT MANY HORMONE REPLACEMENT THERAPIES!
I'M TALKING ABOUT HUSBAND REPLACEMENT TRIALS!

Hormone replacement therapy to help balance hormone levels is an option available to women. Consult with a physician to determine the benefits and risks before starting any treatment.

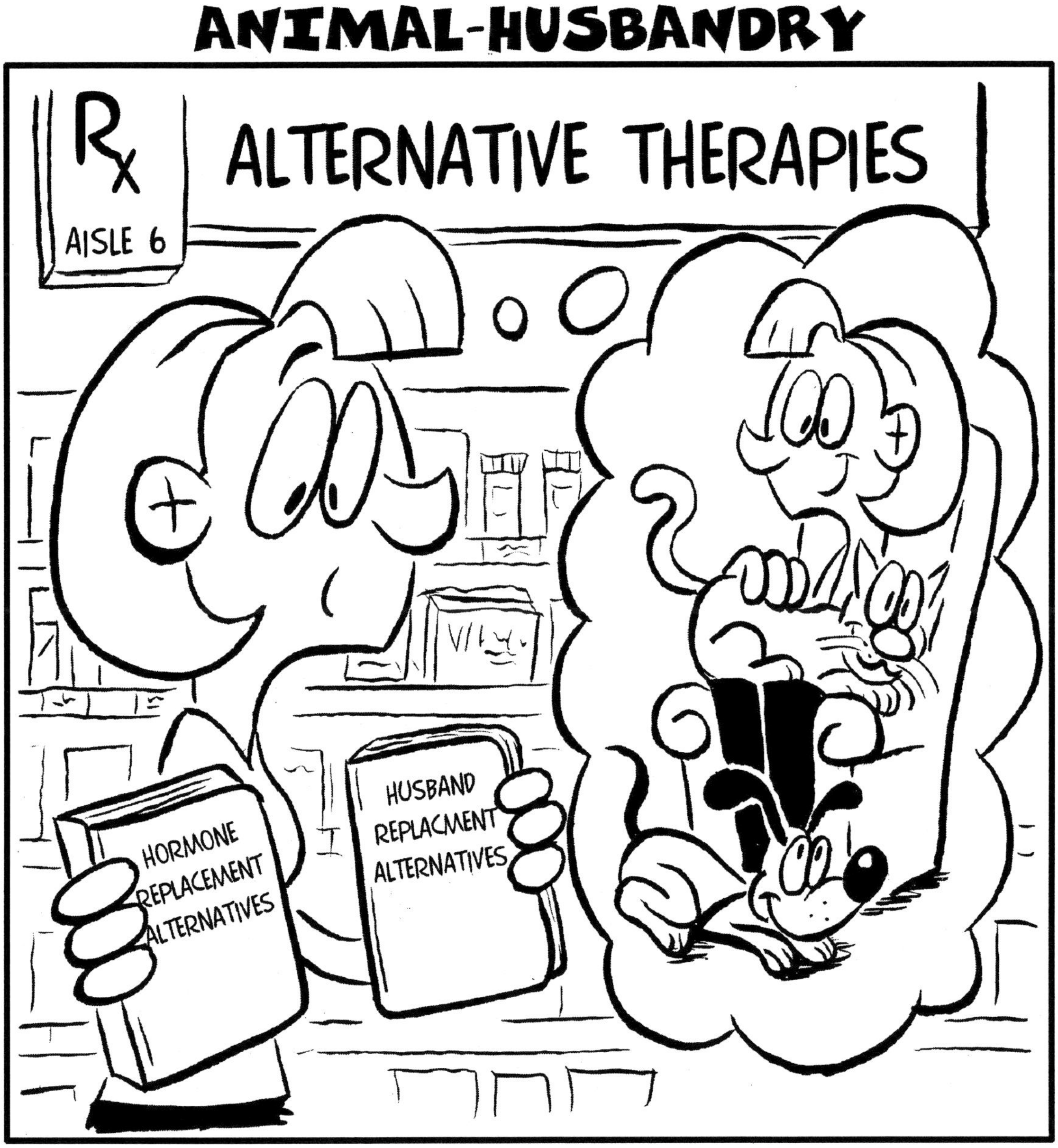

There are alternative therapies for balancing hormone levels including bio-identical hormone therapy and naturally based herbal remedies. Always consult with a physician to determine the benefits and risks before starting any treatment.

THE JOY OF SOY

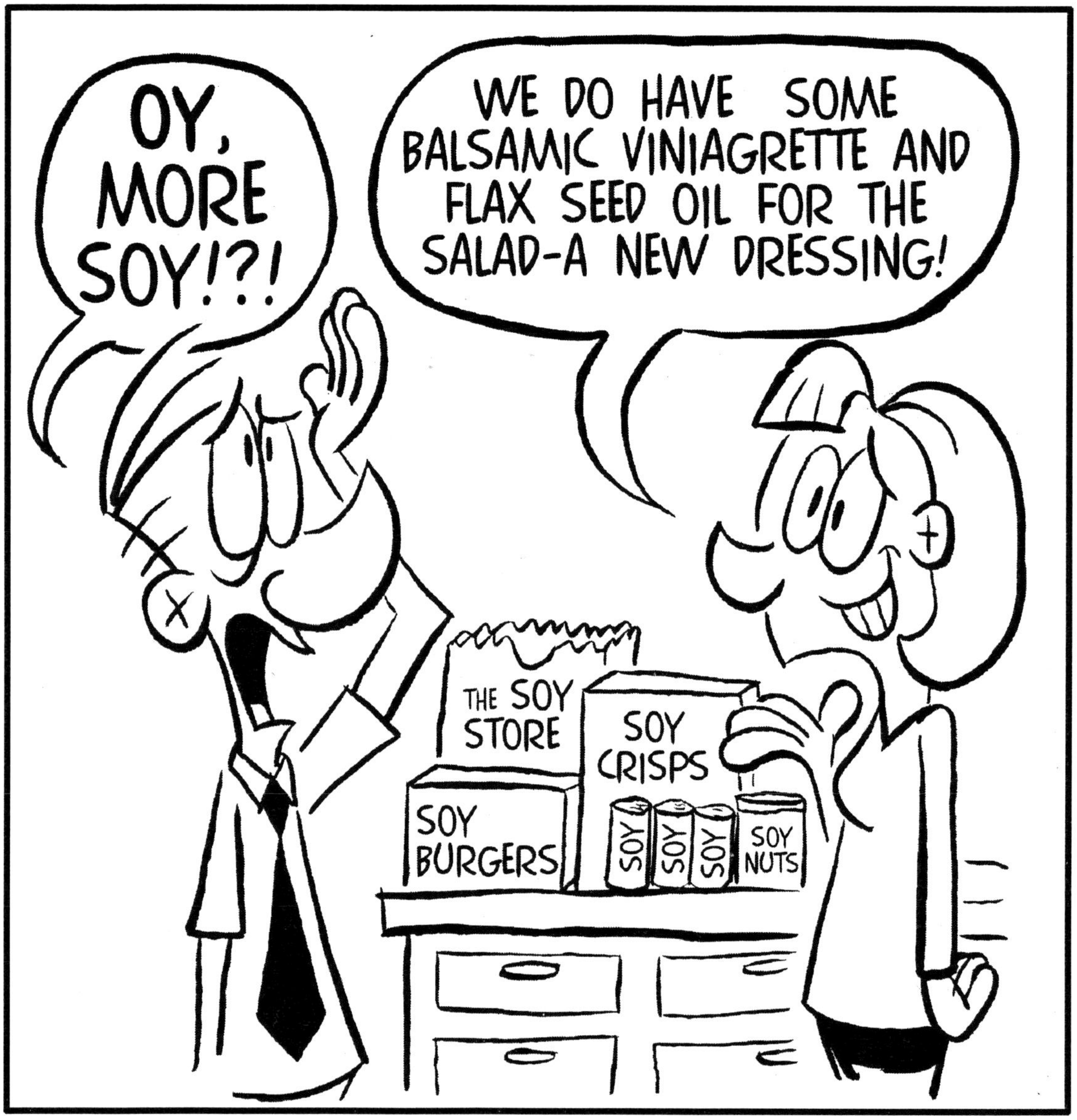
OY, MORE SOY!?!
WE DO HAVE SOME BALSAMIC VINIAGRETTE AND FLAX SEED OIL FOR THE SALAD-A NEW DRESSING!
THE SOY STORE
SOY CRISPS
SOY BURGERS
SOY
SOY
SOY
SOY NUTS

A routine physical exam is recommended every two years including a cholesterol blood test, blood pressure cuff reading, and electrocardiogram to assess heart health. Maintaining healthy body weight is especially important. Food choice, portion size, and exercise all contribute to a healthy heart and overall fitness.

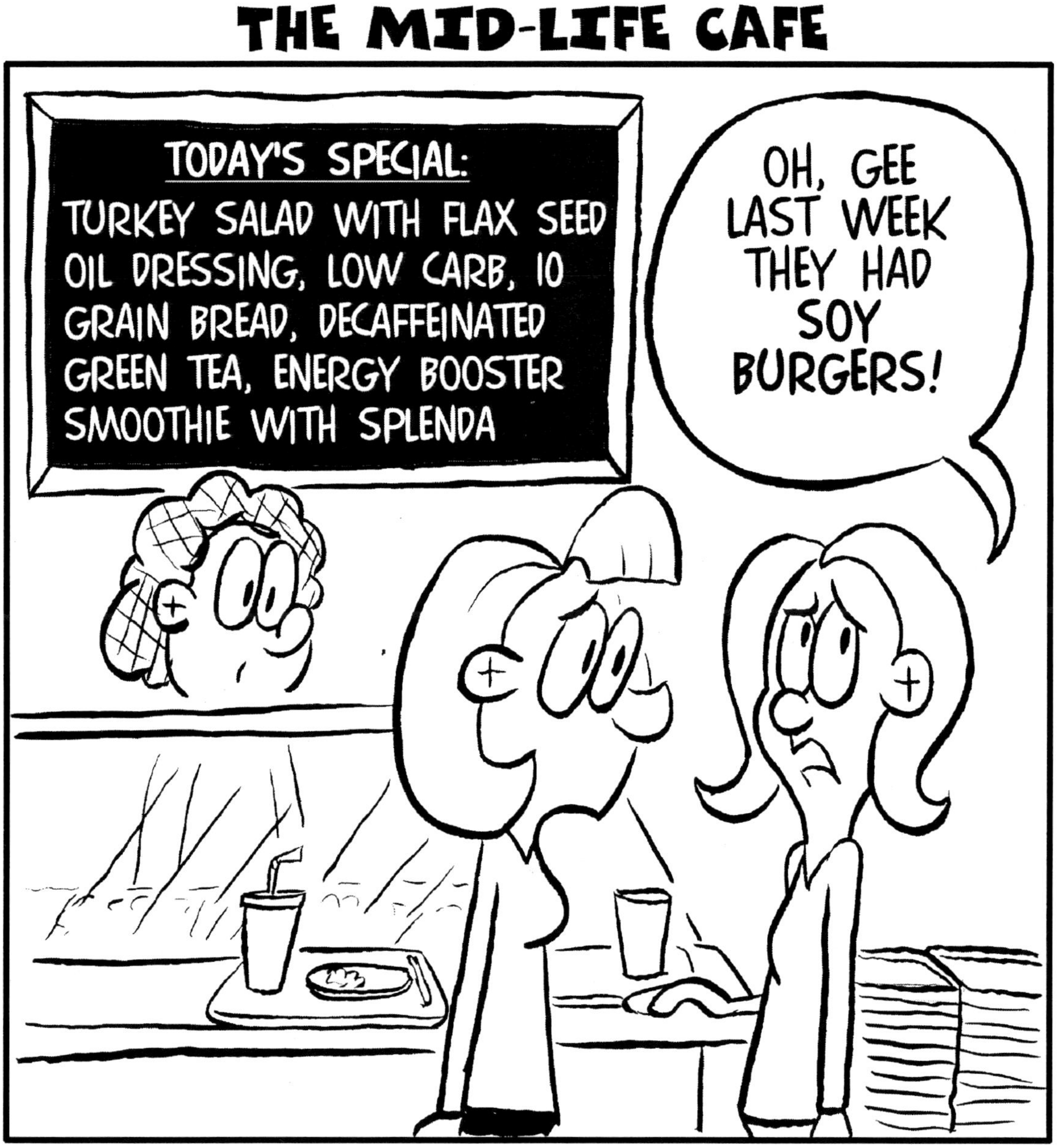
THE MID-LIFE CAFE
TODAY'S SPECIAL:
TURKEY SALAD WITH FLAX SEED OIL DRESSING, LOW CARB, 10 GRAIN BREAD, DECAFFEINATED GREEN TEA, ENERGY BOOSTER SMOOTHIE WITH SPLENDA
OH, GEE LAST WEEK THEY HAD SOY BURGERS!

A diet low in saturated fats is recommended to prevent clogging of the heart arteries. The addition of flax seed oil, whole grain flour and limiting caffeine and sugar intake will help to insure optimal fitness.

MENOPAUSAL MELODIES

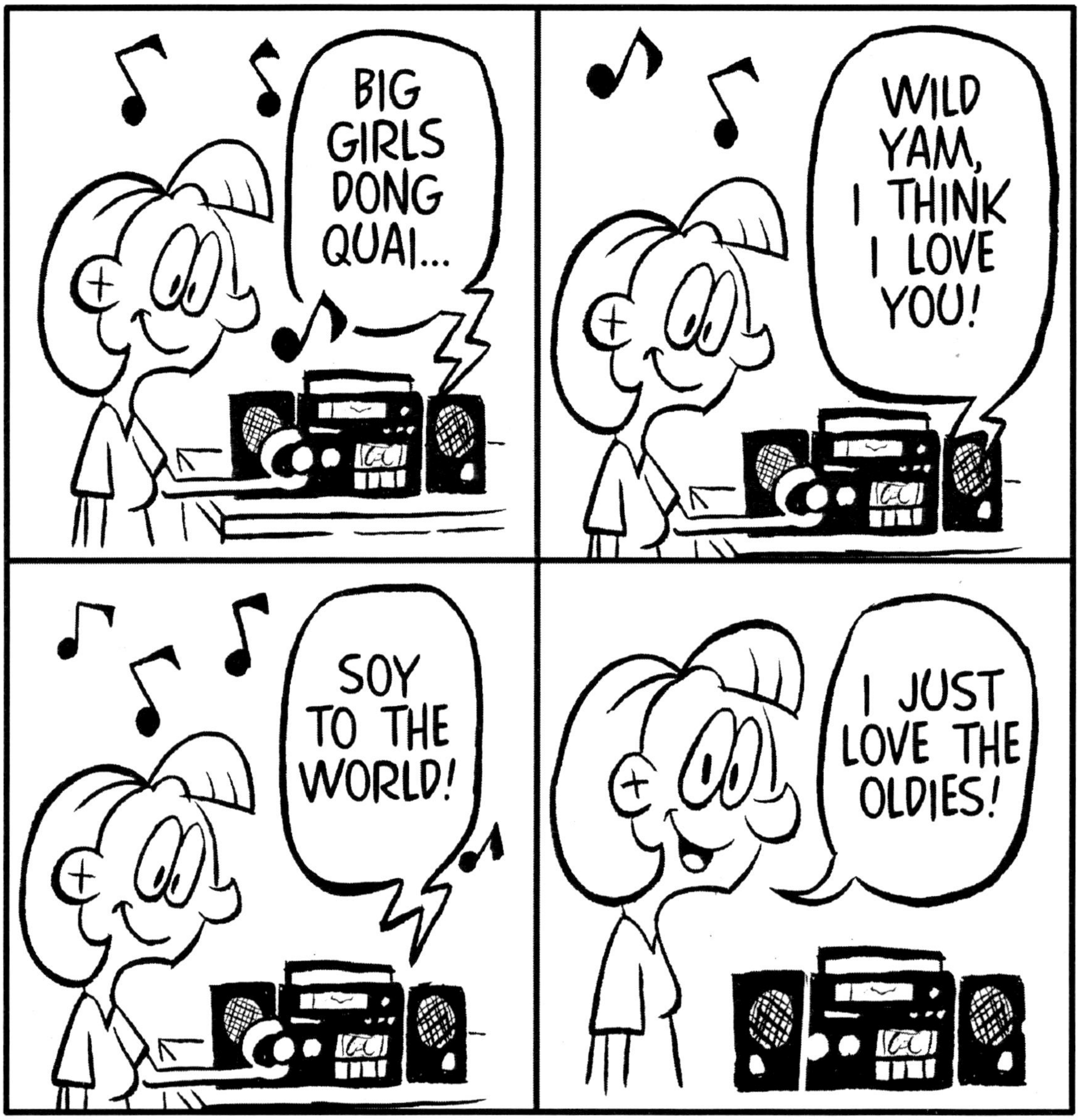
BIG GIRLS DONG QUAI...
WILD YAM, I THINK I LOVE YOU!
SOY TO THE WORLD!
I JUST LOVE THE OLDIES!

Dong Quai, a root herb native to China, has properties that may help to reduce the incidence of hot flashes. Wild Yam and Soy, both plant sources, have been used to mimic hormonal molecules found in the body and to minimize menopausal symptoms.

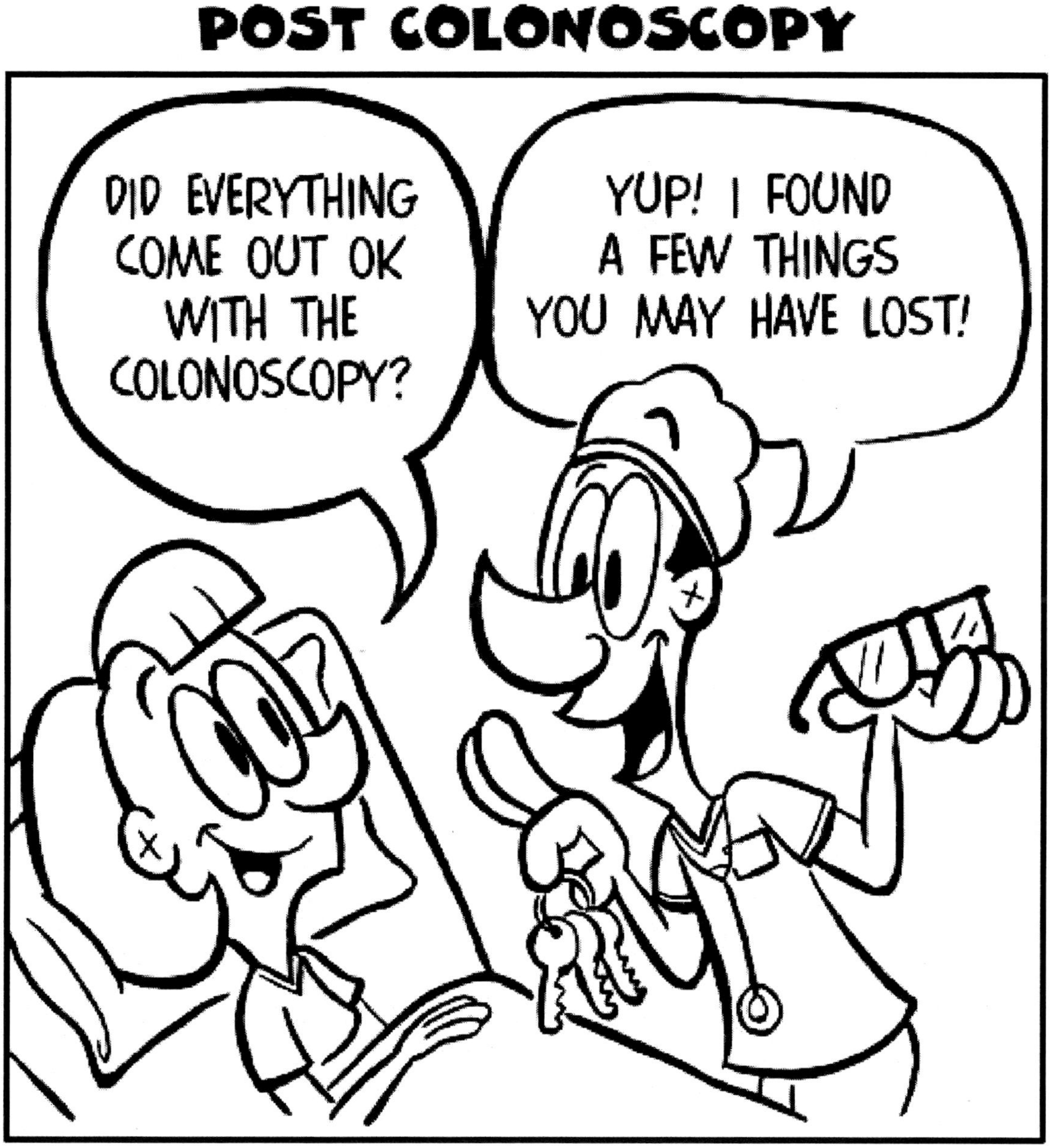
POST COLONOSCOPY
DID EVERYTHING COME OUT OK WITH THE COLONOSCOPY?
YUP! I FOUND A FEW THINGS YOU MAY HAVE LOST!

Beginning at age fifty, a flexible sigmoidoscopy once every five years, or a colonoscopy, once every ten years, is recommended to screen for colorectal cancer, colon polyps, and diverticulitis.

PAP TEST BLUES

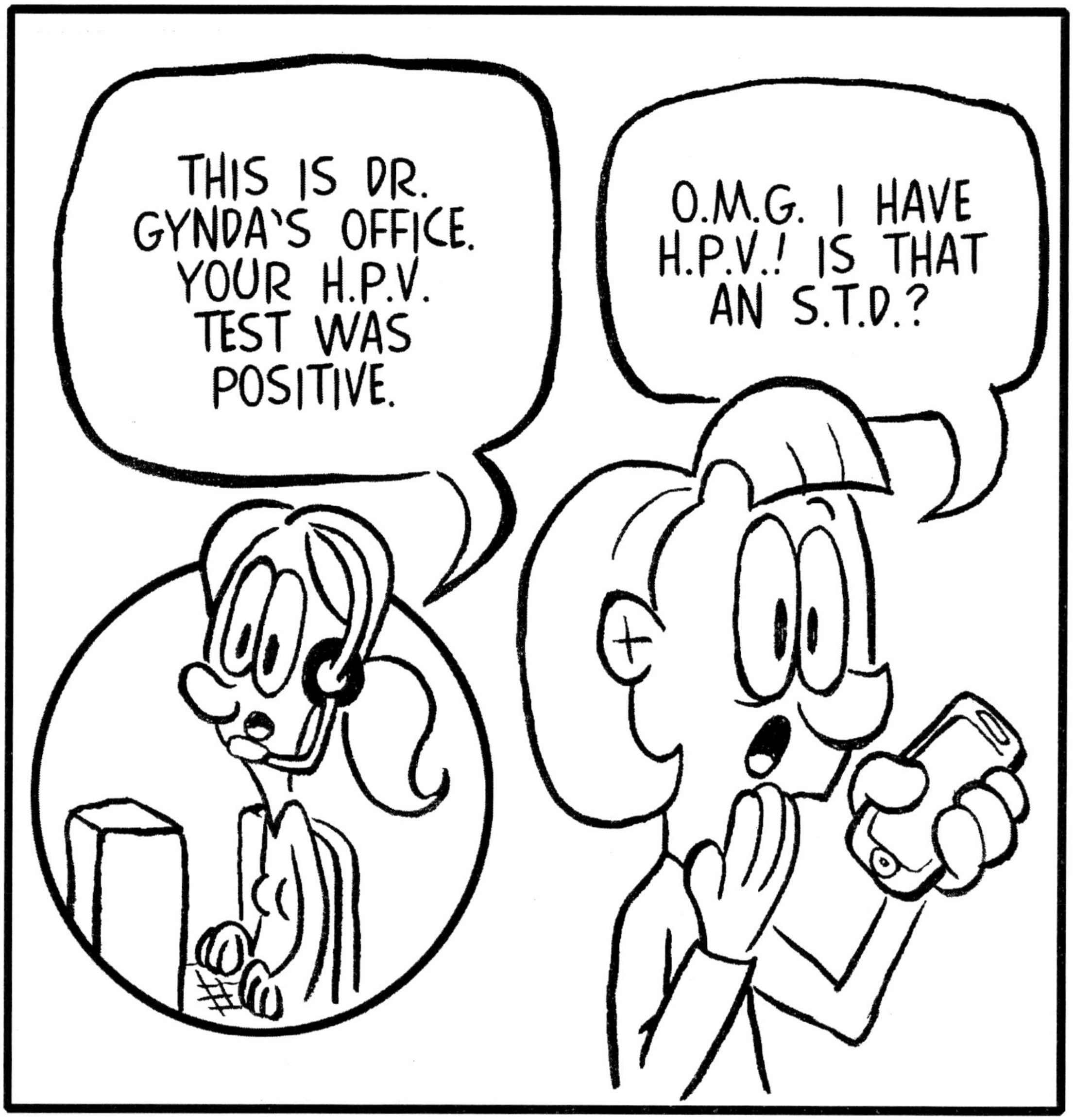
THIS IS DR. GYNDA'S OFFICE. YOUR H.P.V. TEST WAS POSITIVE.
O.M.G. I HAVE H.P.V.! IS THAT AN S.T.D.?

See your gynecologist annually for a breast exam, mammogram, Pap smear, pelvic exam, and Human pappiloma virus (HPV) test. These will screen for breast, ovarian, cervical, and endometrial cancers as well as for sexually transmitted diseases. Although menopause marks the end of childbearing years, a woman is still susceptible to all sexually transmitted diseases.

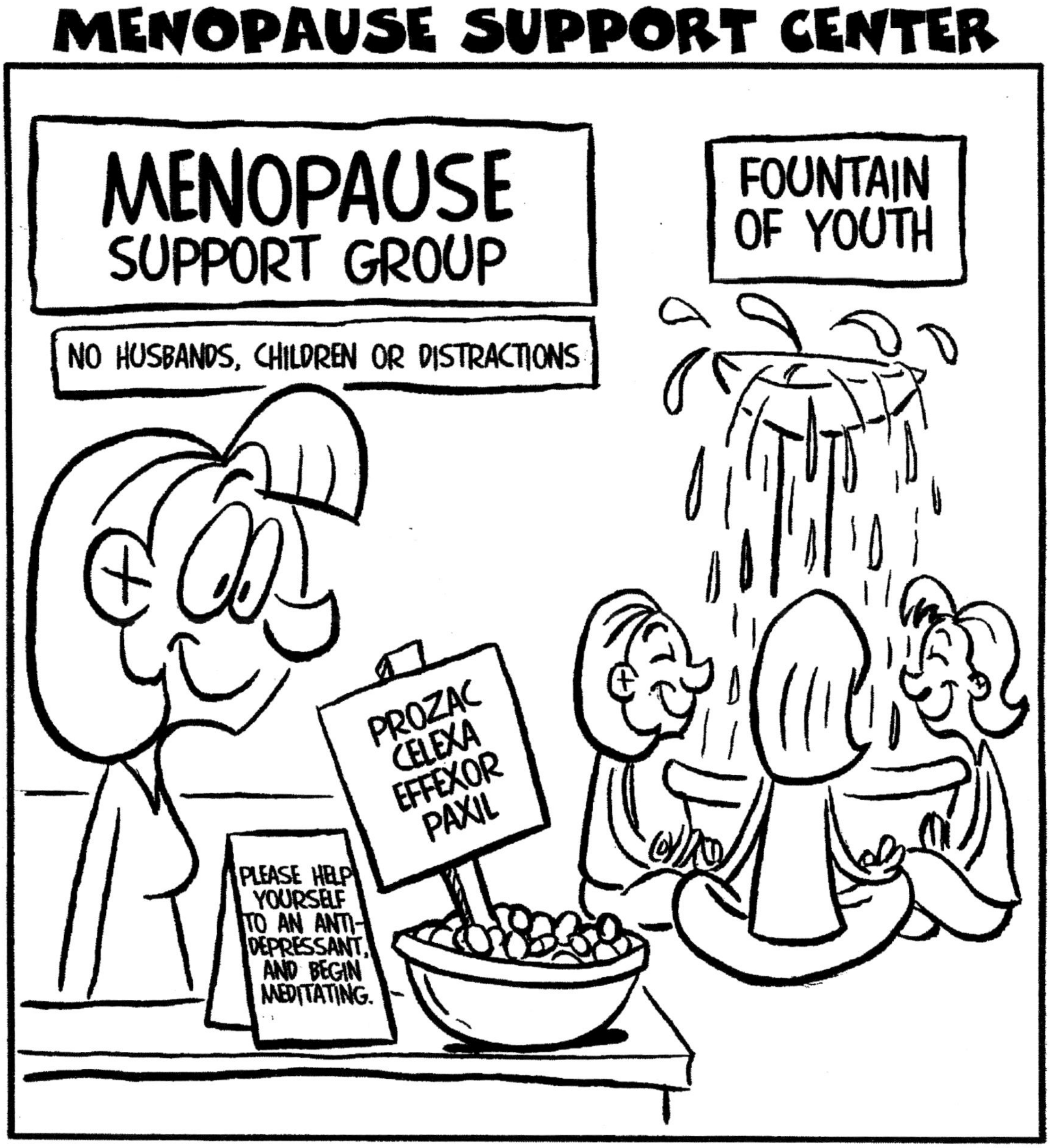
MENOPAUSE SUPPORT CENTER
MENOPAUSE SUPPORT GROUP
NO HUSBANDS, CHILDREN OR DISTRACTIONS
FOUNTAIN OF YOUTH
PROZAC CELEXA EFFEXOR PAXIL
PLEASE HELP YOURSELF TO AN ANTI-DEPRESSANT, AND BEGIN MEDITATING.

Moodiness, anxiety, and depression are common symptoms during the menopausal years. Anti-anxiety and anti-depressant drugs may help to treat these symptoms, but may also have side effects. Exercise, meditation, bio-feedback, yoga, and other breathing exercises are available as natural remedies.

THE VILLAGE WOMEN

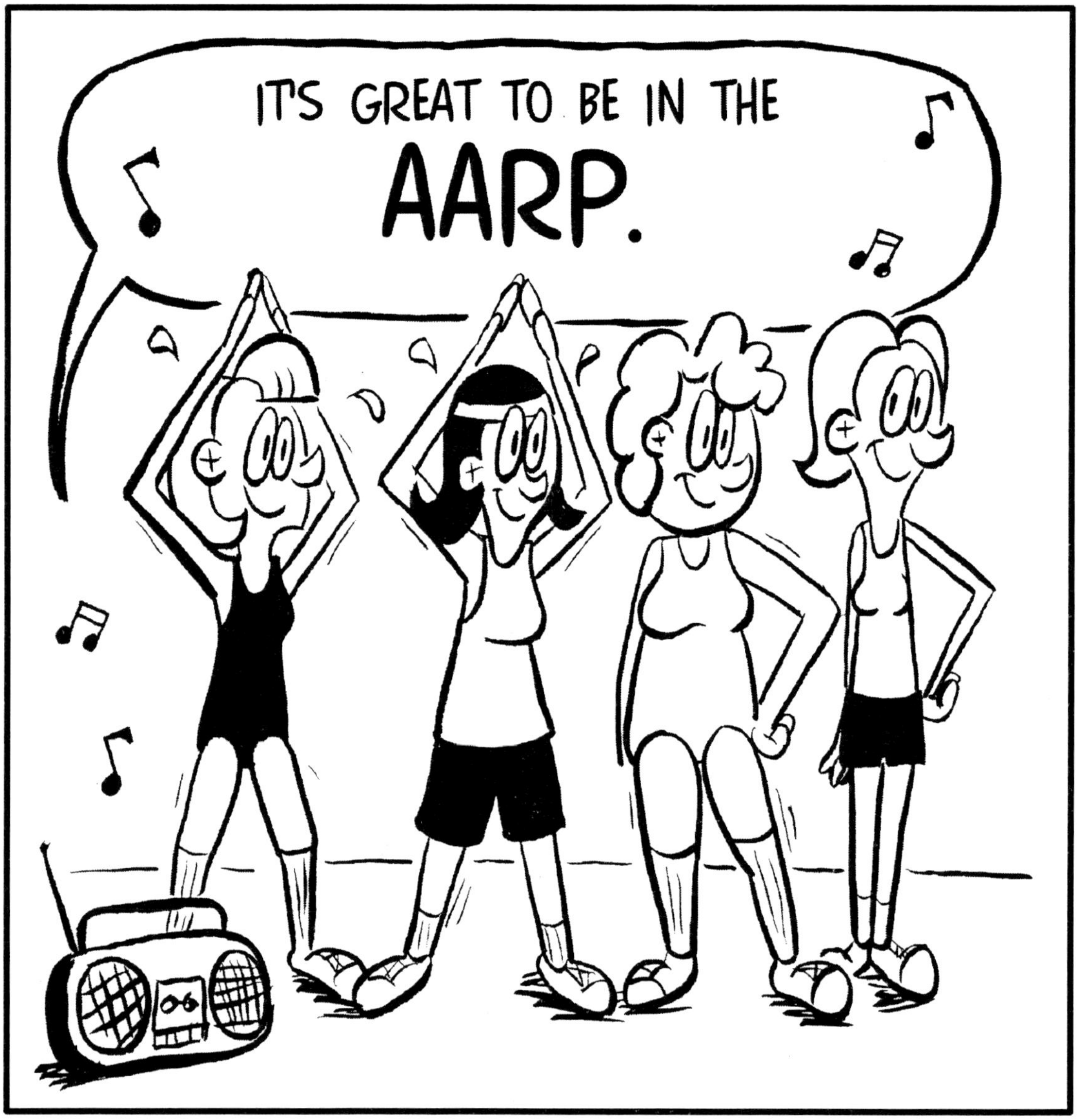

Routine exercise is recommended to prevent all diseases. Current research shows that aerobic exercise helps to improve memory while weight-bearing exercises help to maintain bone density.

THE WHOLE OF ME

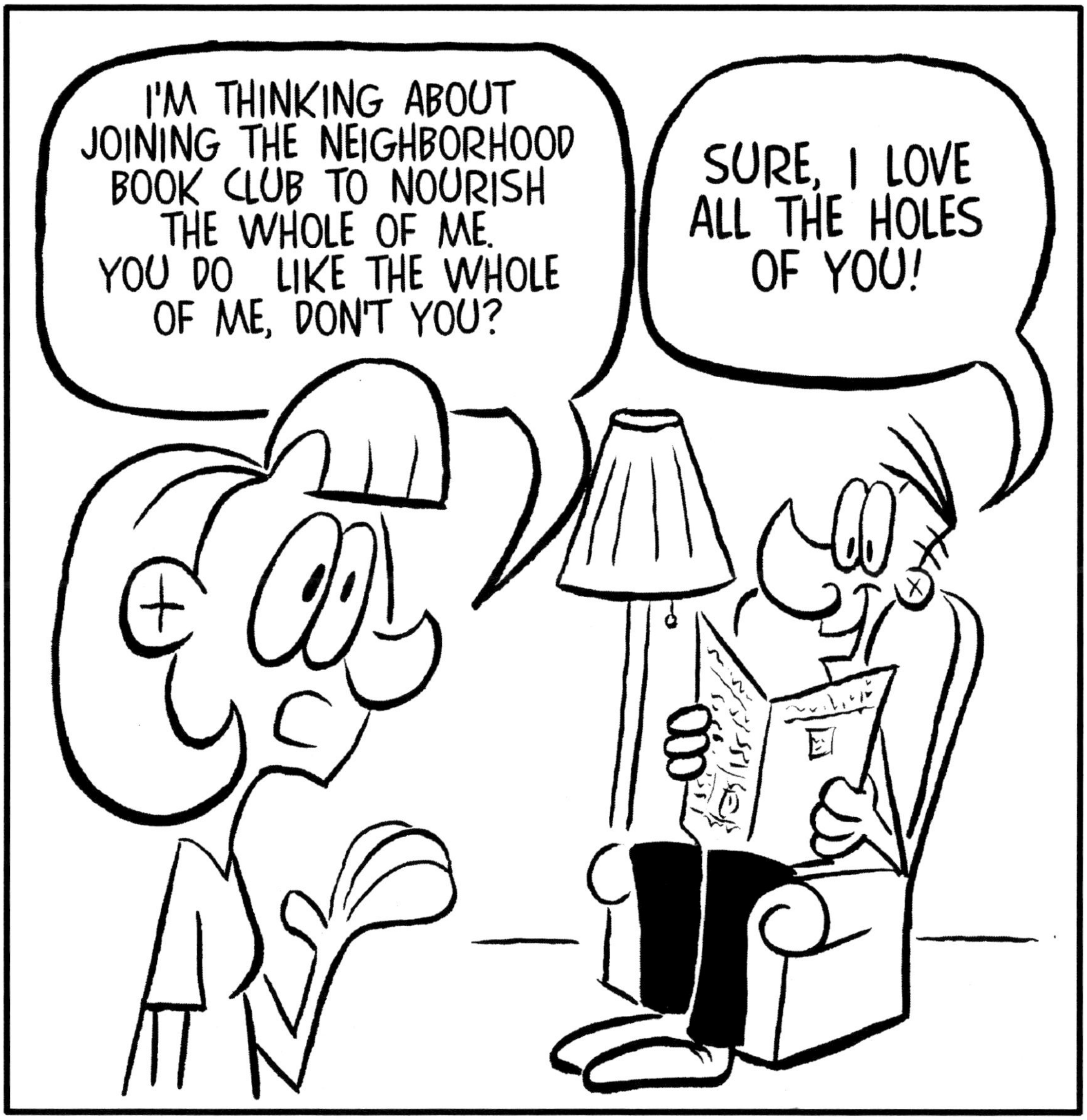
I'M THINKING ABOUT JOINING THE NEIGHBORHOOD BOOK CLUB TO NOURISH THE WHOLE OF ME. YOU DO LIKE THE WHOLE OF ME, DON'T YOU?
SURE, I LOVE ALL THE HOLES OF YOU!

Changes in brain chemistry during menopause point to a greater focus on the "self" at this time. Exploring new areas of interest, developing new hobbies, and pursing enjoyable experiences that nourish your mind and body are helpful ways of making the most of this important transition in your life.

FAMILY COUNSELING

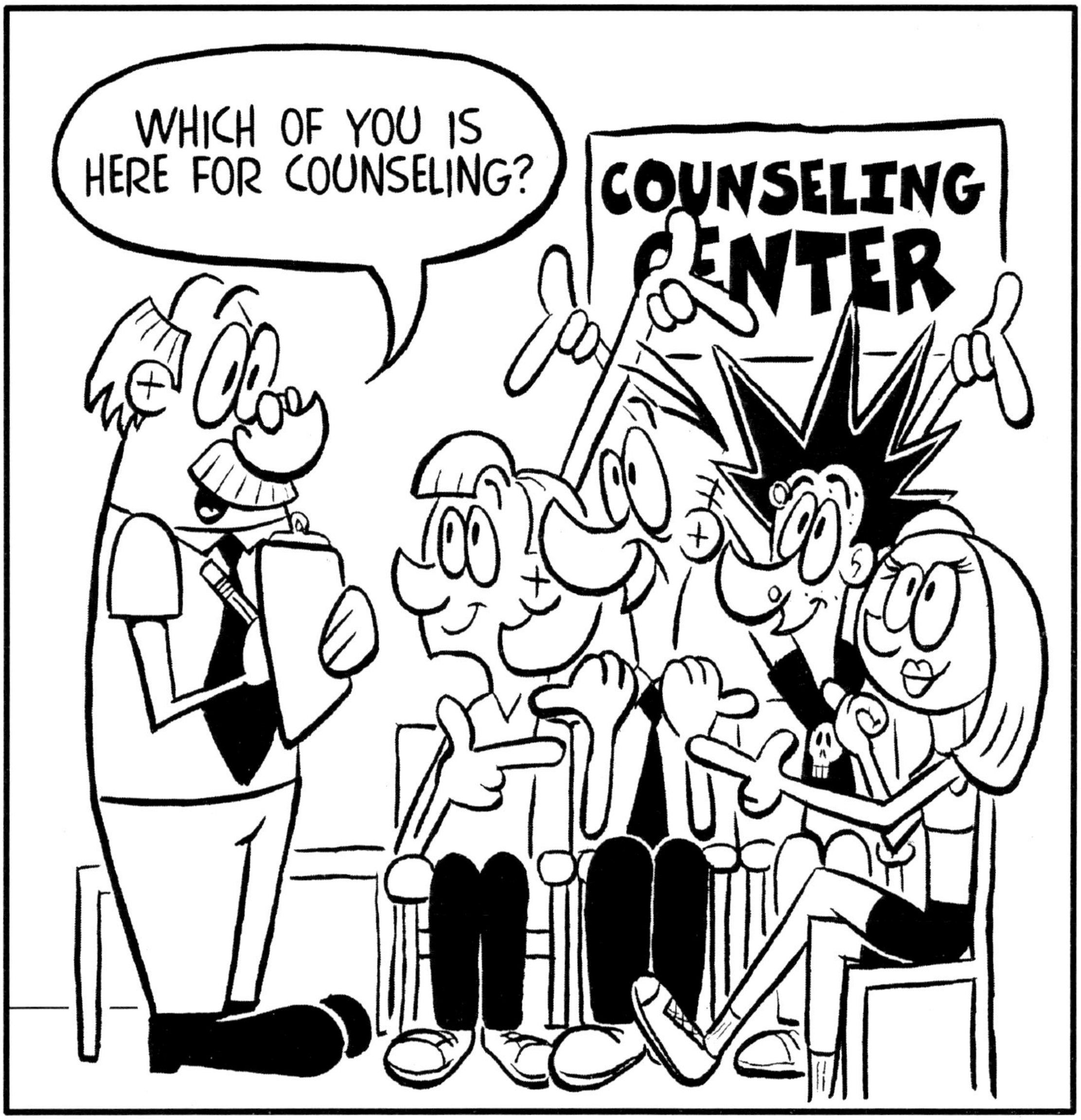

Individual or family counseling during this time of change is another supportive process that may help to address conflicting family needs and to develop healthy coping strategies.

MID-LIFE SCRIPTURE

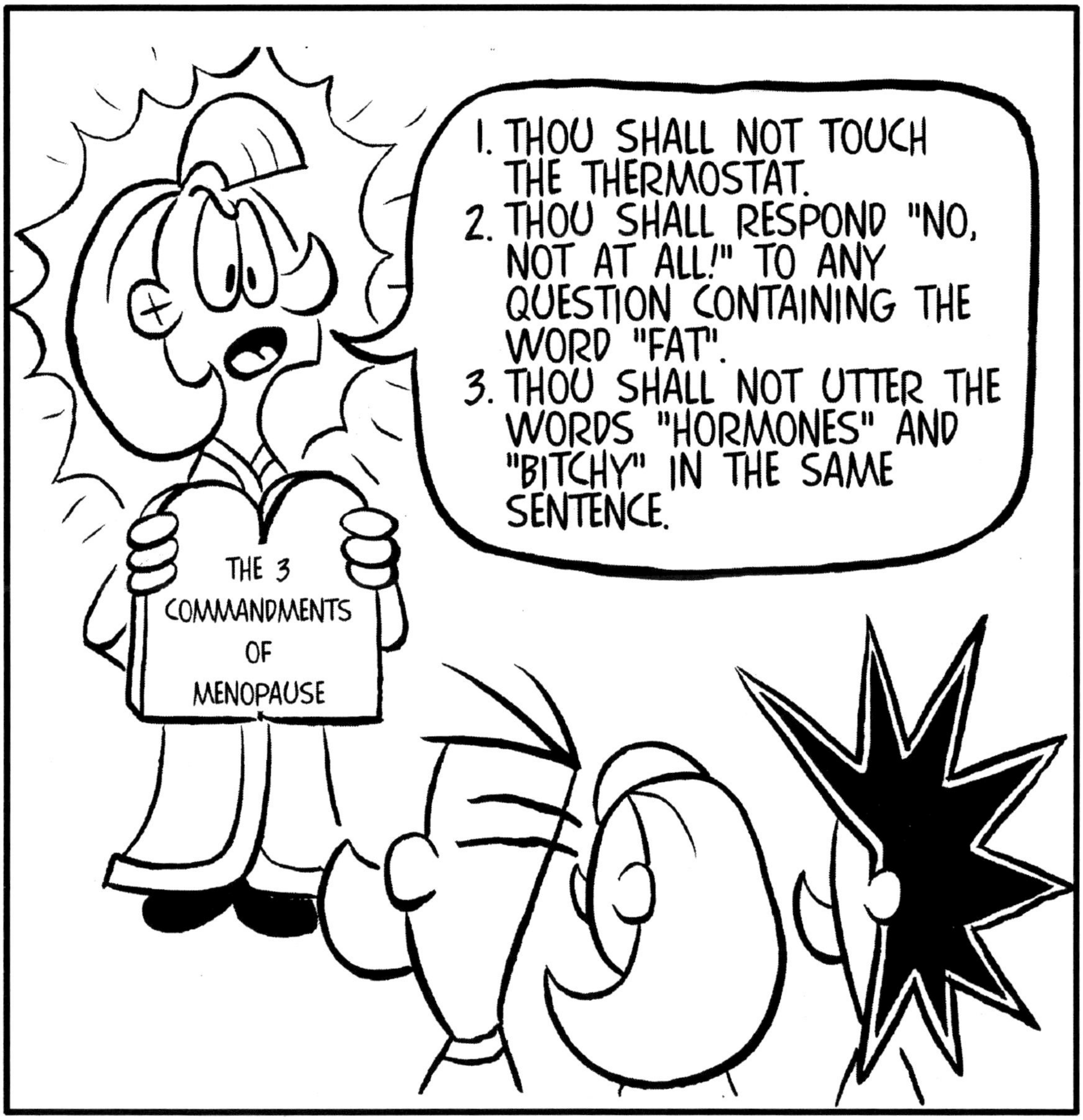
1. THOU SHALL NOT TOUCH THE THERMOSTAT.
2. THOU SHALL RESPOND "NO, NOT AT ALL!" TO ANY QUESTION CONTAINING THE WORD "FAT".
3. THOU SHALL NOT UTTER THE WORDS "HORMONES" AND "BITCHY" IN THE SAME SENTENCE.
THE 3 COMMANDMENTS OF MENOPAUSE

Many women find great comfort in their spirituality as they begin to assess the meaning of their lives.

UPS GROUP

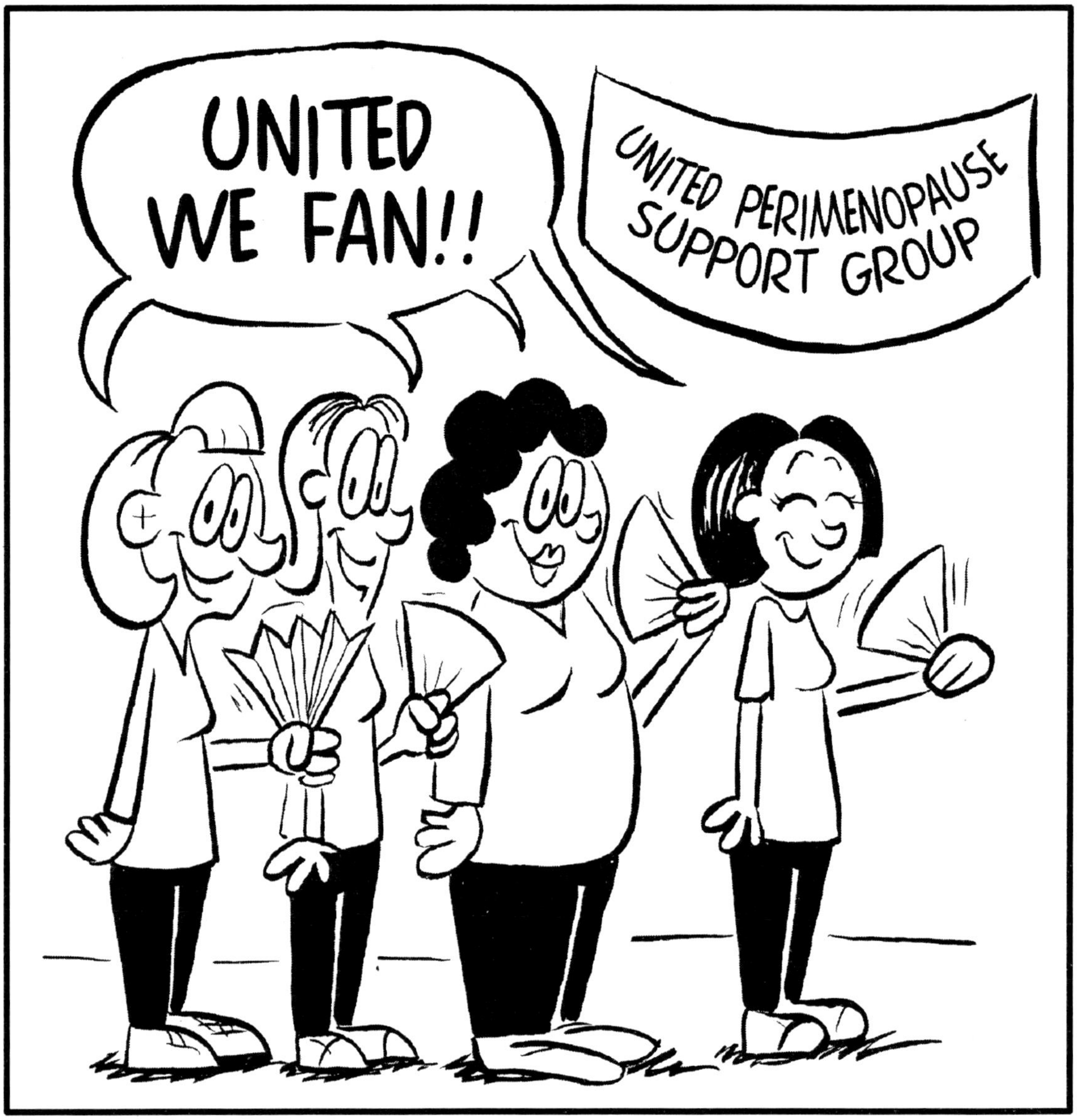

A sympathetic group of women who can relate to these changes may be the best support one can hope to find.

Appendices

Menopause Glossary of Terms

AARP - American Association of Retired Persons.

Anxiety - An unpleasant feeling that is typically associated with uneasiness, apprehension, fear, or worry.

Biofeedback - A technique that trains individuals to improve their health by controlling certain bodily processes that usually happen involuntarily such as heart rate, blood pressure, muscle tension, and skin temperature.

Bioidentical Hormones - Estriol, estradiol, estrone, progesterone, testosterone. These are all synthesized from a plant source (soy or wild yam) to exactly mimic the hormonal molecule found in the body.

Bone Density Scan - An enhanced form of X-ray technology that is used to measure bone mineral density gain or loss.

Bone Mineral Density - Average concentration of minerals in bones.

Breast Exam - A self-inspection of your breasts using your eyes and hands to observe the appearance and feel of your breasts.

Cervical Cancer - Abnormal cells of the cervix or area of the cervix. Human Papillomavirus (HPV) is necessary in the development of almost all cases of cervical cancer.

Cholesterol - A soft, waxy substance found in your bloodstream. Although your body needs cholesterol to help build and maintain cells, too much cholesterol can build up on your artery walls and affect healthy heart functioning.

Colonoscopy - A medical test that allows a physician to perform a visual examination of the inner lining of the large intestine (colon and rectum).

Colon Polyps - Growths in the colon or rectum.

Colorectal Cancer - Abnormal cell growth in the colon or rectum.

Depression - A mental state characterized by feelings of sadness, hopelessness, a sense of inadequacy, or pessimism.

Diverticulitis - An inflammation of the small pouches within the intestinal lining.

Diverticulosis - The condition of having small pouches within the intestinal lining.

Dong Quai (Angelia Sinesis) - Referred to as "female ginseng", the root of this herb, native to China, has proven helpful for relieving hot flashes during menopause. It is also used in the treatment of vaginal dryness and is presumed to increased the effect of ovarian/testicular hormones.

Endometrial Cancer - Abnormal cell formation in the tissue lining of the uterus.

Enzymes - Proteins produced by living cells that function as catalysts in specific biochemical reactions, such as hormone conversion.

Estradiol - A hormone whose level abruptly changes during the menopausal years.

Estrogen - A female hormone that controls sexual development and the menstrual cycle. It also plays an important role in maintaining healthy, strong bones in women. There are three predominant estrogens in a woman's body: estradiol, estriol, and estrone.

Exercise - Body movement is nature's mood modifier and one of the most effective ways of increasing the quality of life for midlife women.

Glucosamine - A drug that aids in pain relief and re-growth of cartilage.

Gynecologist - A medical doctor who diagnoses and treats conditions of the female reproductive system and associated disorders.

Hot Flash - An alteration in thermal stability, which is maintained by the hypothalamus, a brain region located above the pituitary gland on the brain's floor. Estrogen levels manipulate some functions of the hypothalamus. During menopause, as the ovaries produce less estrogen, the hypothalamus senses and responds to the lower estrogen levels by rapidly changing body temperature. The result may be an experience of intense heat and perspiration, typically over the face and neck region.

Heart (Coronary) Arteries - The vessels that deliver oxygen rich blood to the heart.

Hormone - A chemical messenger produced by a gland or organ, that influences a number of metabolic actions in our cells.

Hormone Replacement Therapy (HRT) - One form of medical treatment, typically involving the hormones estrogen, progesterone, and/or testosterone, for women whose hormonal levels have changed due to the menopausal process.

Human Papillomavirus (HPV) - The most common sexually transmitted disease in the United States. It is positively linked to the development of cervical cancer and there is an HPV DNA test available to screen for its presence. There are also vaccinations available for women under the age of 26 years.

Mammogram - An X-ray of the breast.

Methylsulfonylmethane (MSM) - An organic form of sulfer used to relieve pain and inflammation from joints.

Osteoporosis - A condition in which bones become so porous and weak that they are likely to break as a result of a minor injury.

Oxytocin - A mammalian hormone that acts as a neurotransmitter in the brain.

Ovaries - Two glands that produce eggs and sex hormones in women.

Pap Test - A medical test, usually performed by a gynecologist, to take a sample of cells from the cervical area inside of the vagina.

Perimenopause - A period of time when hormonal changes begin to occur in the female body triggering a decrease in estrogen and irregular menstrual cycles.

Progesterone - A female hormone produced by the ovaries. Its function is to prepare the endometrium for egg implantation and to maintain pregnancy. It also serves to balance estrogen.

Resistance Exercise - A type of exercise that uses muscular strength to improve muscle mass, promote energy and support bone density. This type of exercise involves using free weights, wrist weights, exercise bands, and resistance machines found at most gyms and health clubs.

Testosterone -Considered a male hormone, but also produced in smaller quantities by the female body.

Saturated Fats - Fats that consist of triglycerides containing only saturated fatty acid radicals. Examples of foods containing high saturated fats are dairy products, animal fats, and fatty meat. Plant containing saturated fats include coconut, coconut oil, palm oil, and cocoa butter.

Soy - A plant source that is used to mimic the effects of certain hormones in the body and minimize the symptoms of menopause.

Spirituality - The deepest values and meaning by which people live.

Vitamin D - A vitamin formed in the skin when it is exposed to sunlight. Vitamin D helps the body use calcium to help improve bone density. It is available in select foods such as fortified milk, cereals, egg yolks, and fatty fish.

Weight Bearing Exercise - A type of exercise, such as walking or jogging, in which the bones of the legs bear the weight of the body. Weight bearing exercises are helpful for building and keeping bones strong.

Wild Yam - A plant source that is used to mimic the hormonal molecules found in the body and alleviate the symptoms of menopause.

Yoga - A system of physical exercises practiced as part of the Hindu discipline to encourage greater control of the body and mind.

Resources for Women

Women's Health Related Institutes, Foundations, and Associations

Aging

Alliance for Aging Research
2021 K Street NW, Suite 305
Washington, DC 20005
Phone: (202) 293-2856
www.agingresearch.org

National Institute on Aging Information Center (NIAIC)
P.O. Box 8057
Gaithersburg, MD 20898-8057
Phone: (800) 222-2225
www.nia.nih.gov/Health Information/publications

Alternative Medicine

National Center for Complementary and Alternative Medicine
9000 Rockville Pike
Bethesda, MD 20892
www.nccam.nih.gov

Nurture Your Nature
www.nurtureyournature.org

Autoimmune Disease

American Autoimmune Related Diseases Association, Inc.
22100 Gratiot Avenue
East Detroit, MI 48021
Phone: (586) 776-3900
www.aarda.org

American Diabetes Association
1701 North Beauregard Street
Alexandria, VA 22311
Phone: (800) DIABETES
www.diabetes.org

Arthritis Foundation
P.O. Box 7669
Atlanta, GA 30357-0669
Phone: (800) 283-7800
www.arthritis.org

Arthritis and Glucosamine Information Center
www.glucosamine-arthritis.org

Lupus Foundation of America
2000 L Street, NW, Suite 710
Washington, DC 20036
Phone: (202) 349-1155
www.lupus.org

Multiple Sclerosis Association of America
706 Haddonfield Road
Cherry Hill, NJ 08002
Phone: (800) 532-7667
www.msaa.com

The Multiple Sclerosis Foundation, Inc.
6350 North Andrews Avenue
Fort Lauderdale, FL 33309-2130
Phone: (800) 225-6495
www.msfacts.org

National Institute of Arthritis and Musculoskeletal and Skin Diseases
1 AMS Circle
Bethesda, MD 20892-3675
Phone: (877) 226-4267
www.niams.nih.gov

National Institute of Neurological Disorders and Stroke
9000 Rockville Pike
Bethesda, MD 20892
www.nnds.nih.gov

National Multiple Sclerosis Society
733 Third Avenue, 3rd Floor
New York, NY 10017
Phone: (800) 344-4867
www.nationalmssociety.org

Women's Health Related Institutes, Foundations, and Associations

National Organization for Rare Disorders
55 Kenosia Avenue
P.O. Box 1968
Danbury, CT 06813-1968
Phone: (800) 999-6673

Scleroderma Foundation
300 Rosewood Drive, Suite 105
Danvers, MA 01923
Phone: (800) 722-4673
www.scleroderma.org

Sjogrens Syndrome Foundation, Inc.
6707 Democracy Blvd., Suite 325
Bethesda, MD 20817
Phone: (800) 475-6473
www.sjogrens.org

Cancer

American Breast Cancer Foundation
1220 B East Joppa Road, Suite 332
Baltimore, MD 21286
Phone (410) 825-9388
contactABCF@abcf.org
www.abcf.org

American Cancer Society
Phone: (800) ACS-2345
www.cancer.org

American Institute of Cancer Research
1759 R Street NW
Washington, DC 20009
Phone (800) 843-8114
www.aicr.org
Email: aicrweb@aicr.org

American Lung Association
1301 Pennsylvania Ave. NW, Suite 800
Washington, DC 20004
Phone: (202) 785-3355
www.lungusa.org

American Society of Clinical Oncology
2318 Mill Road, Suite 800
Alexandria, VA 22314
Phone (800) 282-2552
Email: membermail@asco.org
www.asco.org

Breast Cancer Network of Strength
1388 Sutter Street, Suite 400
San Francisco, CA 94109-5400
Phone: 415-346-8223
Email: infor@breastcancerfund.org
www.breastcancerfund.org

Breast Cancer Network of Strength
135 S. LaSalle Street, Suite 2000
Chicago, IL 60603
Phone: (312) 986-8338
www.networkofstrength.org

Cancer Care, Inc.
275 Seventh Avenue, Floor 22
New York, NY 10001
Phone: (800) 813-4673
www.cancercare.org

College of American Pathologists
325 Waukegan Road
Northfield, IL 60093-2750
Phone: (800) 323-4040
www.cap.org

Facing Our Risk of Cancer Empowered (FORCE)
16057 Tampa Palms Blvd. W
PMB #373
Tampa, FL 33647
1-866-288-RISK
Email: info@facingourrisk.org
www.facingourrisk.org

Friends for an Earlier Breast Cancer Test
P.O. Box 29524
Greensboro, NC 27429
1-888-792-3062
Email: friends@earlier.org
www.earlier.org

Women's Health Related Institutes, Foundations, and Associations

Gynecologic Cancer Foundation
230 W. Monroe,Suite 2528
Chicago, Il 60606
Phone: (800) 444-4441
www.thegcf.org

HerCancer.com
Phone: (866) HERCANCER
www.hercancer.com

Johns Hopkins Ovarian Cancer Website
1550 Orleans Street, CRB 2, Room 301W
Baltimore, MD 21231
Phone: (410) 614-2905
www.ovariancancer.jhmi.edu

Living Beyond Breast Cancer
Phone: (888) 373-5222
www.lbbc.org

My Health Test Reminder
www.MyHealthTestReminder.com

National Breast Cancer Coalition
1101 17th Street, NW, Suite 1300
Washington, DC 20036
1-800-622-2838
www.stopbreastcancer.org

National Breast Cancer Foundation
2600 Network Blvd., Suite 300
Frisco, Texas 75034
www.nationalbreastcancer.org

National Cancer Institute
Public Inquiries Office
6116 Executive Boulevard, Suite 300
Bethesda, MD 20892-8322
1-800-422-6237
www.cancer.gov

National Cervical Cancer Coalition (NCCC)
6520 Platt Ave. #693
West Hills, CA 91307
1-800-685-5531
www.nccc-online.org

National Cervical Cancer Public Education Campaign
230 W. Monroe, Suite 2528
Chicago, IL 60603
Phone: (312) 578-1439
www.cervicalcancercampaign.org

National HPV and Cervical Cancer Prevention Resource Center American Social Health Association (ASHA)
P.O. Box 13827
Research Traingle Park, NC 27709-3827
Phone: (800) 783-9877

National Lung Cancer Partnership
222 N. Midvale Blvd., Suite 6
Madison, WI 53705
Phone: (608) 233-7905
www.nationallungcancerpartnership.org

Oncology Nursing Society
125 Enterprise Drive
Pittsburgh, PA 15275
Phone: (866) 257-4667
www.ons.org

Ovarian Cancer National Alliance
910 17th Street NW, Suite 1190
Washington, DC 20006
Phone: (866) 399-6262
www.ovariancancer.org

Partnership to End Cervical Cancer
Phone: (212) 798-9753
www.nocervicalcancer.org

Pearl of Wisdom Campaign to Prevent Cervical Cancer
www.pearlofwisdom.us

Susan G. Komen Breast Cancer Foundation
5005 LBJ Freeway, Suite 250
Dallas, TX 75244
Phone: (877) 465-6636
www.komen.org

Tamika & Friends, Inc.
www.tamicaandfriends.org

Women's Health Related Institutes, Foundations, and Associations

Y-Me National Breast Cancer Organization
Phone: (312) 986-8338
www.networkofstrength.org

Cardio/Cerebrovascular Disease

American College of Cardiology
Heart House
2400 North Street NW
Washington, DC 20037
Phone: (800) 253-4636
www.cardiosource.org

American Heart Association
7272 Greenville Avenue
Dallas, TZ 75231
Phone: (800) 242-8721
www.americanheart.org

National Stroke Association
9707 E. Easter Lane, Bldg. B
Centennial, CO 80112
Phone: (800) 787-6537
www.stroke.org

The Hazel K Goddess Fund for Stroke Research in Women
1217 South Flagler Drive, Suite 303
West Palm Beach, FL 33401
Phone: (561) 623-0504
www.thegoddessfund.org

The Heart Truth, National Heart, Lung and Blood Institute
P.O. Box 30105
Bethesda, MD 20824-0105
Phone: (301) 592-8593
www.nhlbi.nih.gov

WomenHeart: The National Coalition for Women with Heart Disease
818 18th Street NW, Suite 1000
Washington, DC 20006
Phone: (877) 771-0030
www.womenheart.org

WomensHearts.org
www.womenshearts.org

Chronic Pain

National Vulvodynia Association
P.O. Box 4491
Silver Spring, MD 20914-4491
Phone: (301) 299-0775
www.nva.org

Diabetes

National Diabetes Education Program
One Diabetes Way
Bethesda, MD 20814-9692
Phone: (301) 496-3583
www.ndep.nih.gov

Endocrinology

American Thyroid Association
6066 Leesburg Pike, Suite 550
Falls Church, VA 22041
Phone: (703) 998-8893
www.thyroid.org

The Hormone Foundation/The Endocrine Society
8401 Connecticut Ave., Suite 900
Chevy Chase, MD 20815-5817
Phone: (800) HORMONE
www.hormone.org

Women's Health Related Institutes, Foundations, and Associations

Fibromyalgia

National Fibromyalgia Association
2121 S. Towne Centre Place,
Suite 300
Anaheim, CA 92806
Phone: (714) 921-0150
www.fmaware.org

National Fibromyalgia Research Association
www.nfra.net

Fitness/Physical Therapy

American Council for Fitness and Nutrition
1350 1 Street, Suite 300
Washington, DC 20005
www.acfn.org

National Women's Health Information Center
U.S. Department of Health and Human Services
Office on Women's Health
Physical Activity
Phone: (800) 994-9662
www.womenshealth.gov

The Section on Women's Health of the American Physical Therapy Association
111 Fairfax Avenue
Alexandria, VA 22314
Phone: (800) 999-APTA X3229
www.womenshealthapta.org

General & Internal Medicine

American Medical Association
515 North State Street
Chicago, IL 60654
1-800-621-8335
www.ama-assn.org

American Osteopathic Association
142 East Ontario Street
Chicago, Il 60661
Phone: (800) 621-1773
www.osteopathic.org

National Anemia Action Council
555 E. Wells Street, Suite 1100
Milwaukee, WI 53202
Phone: (414) 225-0138
www.anemia.org

Intersticial Cystitis Association
100 Park Avenue, Suite 108A
Rockville, MD 20850
www.ichelp.org

Headaches

National Headache Foundation
820 N. Orleans, Suite 217
Chicago, IL 60610
Phone: (888) NHF-5552
www.headaches.org

Infectious Diseases

Spotlight on Shingles
www.spotlightonshingles.com

Menopause

American Menopause Foundation
866 United Nations Plaza
Suite 508
New York, NY 10017
www.americanmeopause.org

Asia Pacific Menopause Federation
Dept of Obsetrics and Gynaecology
The Prince of Wales Hospital Shatin, NT
Hong Kong SAR China
852-26322800
Email: info@apmf.net

Women's Health Related Institutes, Foundations, and Associations

Austrlian Menopause Society
P.O. Box 1228
Bluderim Qld 4556
Australia
617-4642 1603

European Menopause and Andropause Society (EMAS)
c/o Kenes International
P.O. Box 1726
1-3, rue de Chantepoulet
CH-1211 Geneva 1
Switzerland
+41 22 906 91 74
Email: infor@emasonline.org

International Menopause Society
P.O. Box 687
Wray
Lancaster
LA2 8WY
UK
+44 1524221190
Email: jwright.ims@btopenworld.com

International Premature Ovarian Failure Association
P.O. Box 23643
Alexandria, VA 22304
703-913-4787
Email: membersupport@popsupport.org

Japan Menopause Society
c/o Congress Corporation
Kohsai-kaikan Bldg.
5-1 Kojimachi
Chiyoda-ku
Tokyo 102-8481
Japan
+81-3-3263-4035
Email: jms@congre.co.jp

North American Menopause Society
5900 Landerbrook Drive, Suite 390
Mayfield Heights, OH 44124
Phone: 440-442-7550
www.menopause.org

Musculoskeletal Health

American Academy of Orthopaedic Surgeons
6300 North River Road
Rosemont, IL 60018-4212
Phone: (847) 823-7186

American Bone Health
1814 Franklin Street, Suite 620
Oakland, CA 94612
Phone: (888) 843-9391
www.americanbonehealth.org

American College of Rheumatology
2200 Lake Boulevard NE
Atlanta, GA 30319
Phone: (404) 633-3777
www.rheumatology.org

International Osteoporosis Foundation
9, rue Juste-Olivier
CH-1260 Nyon
Switzerland
Phone: +41 22 994 0100

National Institute of Arthritis and Musculoskeletal and Skin Diseases
2 AMS Circle
Bethesda, MD 20892-3676
Phone: (800) 624-BONE
www.niams.nih.gov

National Osteoporosis Foundation (NOF)
1150 17th Street NW, Suite 850
Washington, DC 20036-4644
Phone (800) 223-9994
www.nof.org

NIH Osteoporosis and Related Bone Diseases
National Resource Center
2 AMS Circle
Bethesda, MD 20892-3676
Phone (800) 624-2663
www.niams.nig.gov/Health_Infor/bone/default.asp

Women's Health Related Institutes, Foundations, and Associations

Neurology and Mental Health

Alzheimer's Association
225 N. Michigan Avenue, Floor 17
Chicago, IL 60601-7633
Phone: (800) 272-3900
www.alz.org

Anxiety Disorders Association of America
8730 Georgia Avenue
Silver Springs, MD 20910
Phone: (240) 485-1001
www.adaa.org

American Parkinson Disease Association
www.apdaparkinson.com

American Psychiatric Association
1000 Wilson Blvd., Suite 1825
Arlington, VA 22209
Phone: (888) 35-PSYCH
www.healthyminds.org

American Psychological Association
750 First Street NE
Washington, DC 20002-4242
Phone: (800) 374-2721
www.apa.org

Center for Women's Mental Health
185 Cambridge Street, Suite 2200
Boston, MA 02114
Phone: (617) 724-7792

Depression and Related Affective Disorders Association
8201 Greensboro Drive, Suite 300
McLean, VA 22102
www.drada.org

Epilepsy Foundation
8301 Professional Place
Landover, MD 20785
Phone: (800) 332-1000
www.epilepsyfoundation.org

For Grace
605 W. Olympic Blvd., Suite 800
Los Angeles, CA 90015
Phone: (818) 760-7635
www.forgrace.org

National Institute of Mental Health
6001 Executive Blvd., Room 8184, MSC 9663
Bethesda, MD 20892-9663
Phone: (866) 615-6464
www.nimh.nih.gov

National Mental Health Association
2000 N. Beauregard Street, 6th Floor
Alexandria, VA 22311
Phone: (703) 684-7722
www.nmha.org

National Alliance for the Mentally Ill
3803 Fairfax Drive, Suite 100
Arlington, VA 22203
Phone: (703) 524-7600
www.nami.org

Substance Abuse & Mental Health Services Administration
P.O. Box 2345
Rockville, MD 20847-2345
Phone: (877) 726-4727
www.samhsa.gov

Women's Behavioral Healthcare
Western Psychiatric Institute and Clinic
3811 O'Hara Street
Pittsburgh, PA 15213
Phone: (800) 436-2461

Women's Health Interactive
9654 W. 131st Street, Suite 411
Palos Park, IL 60464
www.womens-health.com

Women's Health Related Institutes, Foundations, and Associations

Nutrition

American Dietetic Association
120 South Riverside Plaza, Suite 2000
Chicago, IL 60606-6995
Phone: (800) 877-1600
www.eatright.org

National Association of Nutrition Professionals
P.O. Box 1884
Rancho Cordova, CA 95741
Phone: (800) 342-8037
www.nanp.org

Obesity, Eating Disorders, Metabolism

National Institute of Diabetes and Digestive and Kidney Diseases
Building 31, Room 9A06
31 Center Drive, MSC 2560
Bethesda, MD 20892-2560
Phone: (301) 496-3583
www.niddk.nih.gov

National Lipedema Association
www.lipedema.org

Reproductive Health

American College of Obstetricians and Gynecologists (ACOG)
P.O. Box 96920
Washington, DC 20090-6920
Phone (202) 638-5577
www.acog.org

American College of Nurse-Midwives
8403 Crossville Road, Suite 1550
Silver Springs, MD 20910
Phone: (240) 485-1800
www.midwife.org

American Society for Reproductive Medicine
1209 Montgomery Highway
Birmingham, AL 35216-2809
Phone: (205) 978-5000
www.asrm.org

Association of Reproductive Health Professionals
1901 L Street NW, Suite 300
Washington, DC 20036
Phone (202) 466-3825
www.arhp.org

Planned Parenthood Federation of America
434 West 33rd Street
New York, NY 10001
Phone: (212) 541-7800
www.plannedparenthood.org

Resolve: The National Infertility Association
1760 Old Meadow Road, Suite 500
McLean, VA 22102
Phone: (703) 556-7172
www.resolve.org

Sexual Health

Sex Brain Body: Make the Connection
Phone: (212) 880-5258
www.sexbrainbody.com

The Women's Sexual Health Foundation
www.twshf.org

Sexually Transmitted Diseases

American Social Health Association
P.O. Box 13827
Research Triangle Park, NC 27709
Phone: (919) 361-8400
www.ashastd.org

Women's Health Related Institutes, Foundations, and Associations

National Institute of Allergy and Infectious Diseases
6610 Rockledge Drive, MSC 6612
Bethesda, MD 20892-6612
Phone: (866) 284-4107
www.niaid.nih.gov

STD Information
CDC-INFO
Contact Center
Phone (800) 232-4636
Email: cdcinfo@cdc.gov

United Nations Development Fund for Women
304 East 45th Street, 15th Floor
New York, NY 10017
Phone: (212) 906-6400
www.genderandaids.org

HIV/AIDS

AIDS Action
1730 M Street NW, Suite 611
Washington, DC 20036
Phone: (202) 530-8030
www.aidsaction.org

AIDS Clinical Trials Information Source
www.actis.org

American Foundation for AIDS Research
120 Wall Street, 13th Floor
New York, NY 10005-3908
Phone: (212) 806-1600
www.amfar.org

Know HIV AIDS.org
P.O. Box 6003
Rockville, MD 20849-6003
Phone: (800) 458-5231
www.hivtest.org

National Association of People with AIDS
8401 Colesville Road, Suite 505
Silver Spring, MD 20910
Phone: (240) 247-0880
www.napwa.org

Project Inform
1375 Mission Street
San Francisco, CA 94103-2621
Phone: (415) 558-8669
www.projinf.org

Additional Health Resources for Women

Black Women's Health Imperative
1726 M Street, NW, Suite 300
Washington, CD 20036
Phone: (202) 548-4000
www.blackwomenshealth.org

CDC National Prevention Information Network (NPIN)
P.O. Box 6003
Rockville, MD 20849-6003
1-800-458-5231
Email: infor@cdcnpin.org

CDC- Women's Health
1600 Clifton Road
Atlanta, GA 30333
Phone: (800) 232-4636

Getting Better
www.getbetterhealth.com

Hadassah, the Women's Zionist Organization of America, Inc.
Kiryat Hadassah
p.o.b. 12000
91120 Jerusalem
Israel
Phone: (02) 6777111
www.hadassah.org

Women's Health Related Institutes, Foundations, and Associations

Jean Hailes Foundation for Women's Health
173 Carinish Road
Clayton, VIC 3168
1 800 151 441
Email: education@jeanhailes.org.au

National Institute of Health
9000 Rockville Pike
Bethesda, MD 20892
Phone: (301) 496-4000
www.nih.gov

National Library of Medicine's Health Services/Technology Assessment Text
www.ncbi.nlm.nih.gov

National Women's Health Information Center
U.S. Dept. of Health and Human Services
Office on Women's Health
Washington, DC 20036
Phone: (800) 994-9662
www.4women.gov

National Women's Health Resource Center
157 Broad Street, Suite 106
Red Bank, NJ 07701
Phone: (877) 986-9472
www.healthywomen.org

Nurse Practitioners in Women's Health
505 C Street, Northeast
Washington, DC 20002
Phone: (202) 543-9693
www.npwh.org

Patient Advocate Foundation
421 Butler Farm Road
Hampton, VA 23666
Phone: (800) 532-5274

Society for Women's Health Research
1025 Connecticut Ave Nw, Suite 701
Washington, DC 20036
202-223-8224
Email: info@swhr.org
www.womenshealthreseach.org

The Daisy Network
P.O. Box 183
Rossendale
BB4 6WZ
UK

The Uplift Community Foundation
Phone: (202) 785-0022
www.upliftfoundation.org

Washington Women in Need
2285 116th Avenue NE, Suite 100
Bellevue, WA 98004
424-451-8845
www.wawomeninneed.org

Women to Women
3 Marina Road
Yarmouth, Maine 04096
1-207-846-6163
www.womentowomen.com

For additional information about popular midlife websites, blogs and on-line communities, visit www.hotflashesforwomen.com

About The Author

Robin L. Gordon. M.A., M.S.W.

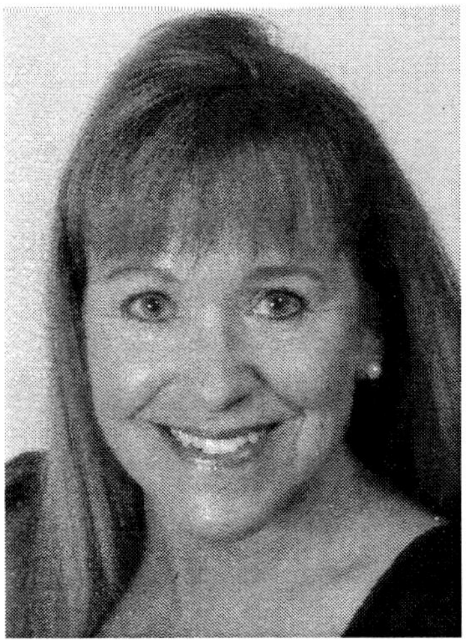

Robin L. Gordon is a menopausal wife and mother. As a writer and illustrator, she injects humor and humanity into her work to help people through various life passages. Robin's most recent book, **"Hot Flashes: Marriage and Motherhood in the Menopausal Years**" is her way to humorously share some life-changing information about this challenging and unique period in a woman's life. She is a well recognized speaker and shares her research and humor in a multi-media presentation entitled "***Hot Flashes for Women of a Certain Age***". She is also the founder of the busy website**, hotflashesforwomen.com**, committed to health education and inspiration.

A graduate of the University of Michigan with Masters degrees in Social Work and Special Education, Robin also maintains certification in Human Resource Development and Training. She has had a successful career as an educator, state education consultant, speaker, trainer, author, illustrator and mediator.

Committed to create inspirational work for all ages and stages, Robin is also an author/illustrator of the children's book, "**Peaceful Thoughts**" and "**Lift: A Gosling's First Flight**".

Robin is happily married and still coping with the "hot flashes", a gift from the sun gods!

Contact the author for additional information about speaking to large groups with her multi-media presentation, "***Hot Flashes for Women***".

www.hotflashesforwomen.com or rktpeaceful@yahoo.com or

robin@hotflashesforwomen.com.

Would you like to get a copy for someone you care about?

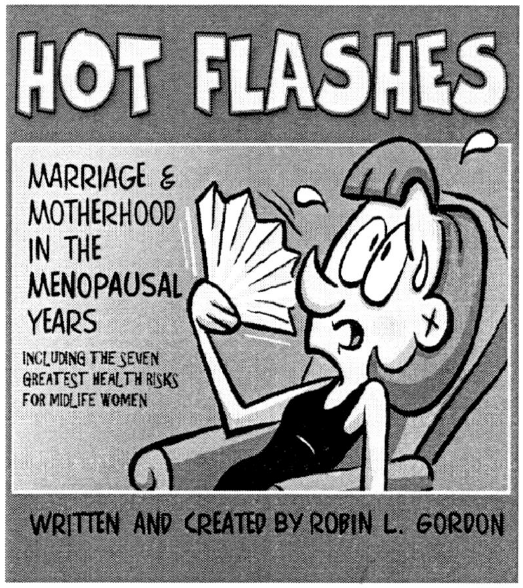

Please go to

www.hotflashesforwomen.com

or contact the author at

rktpeaceful@yahoo.com or

robin@hotflashesforwomen.com

A portion of the proceeds from the sale of this book are donated to a variety of women's healthcare organizations.